Cloud-based Solutions
for Healthcare IT

Cloud-based Solutions for Healthcare IT

A.K. Soman, *Ph.D.*

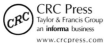

CRC Press
Taylor & Francis Group
an **informa** business
www.crcpress.com

6000 Broken Sound Parkway, NW
Suite 300, Boca Raton, FL 33487
270 Madison Avenue
New York, NY 10016
2 Park Square, Milton Park
Abingdon, Oxon OX 14 4RN, UK

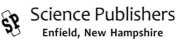

Science Publishers
Enfield, New Hampshire

Published by Science Publishers, P.O. Box 699, Enfield, NH 03748, USA
An imprint of Edenbridge Ltd., British Channel Islands

Email: _info@scipub.net_   Website: _www.scipub.net_

Marketed and distributed by:

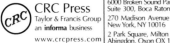

	6000 Broken Sound Parkway, NW
CRC Press	Suite 300, Boca Raton, FL 33487
Taylor & Francis Group	270 Madison Avenue
an **informa** business	New York, NY 10016
	2 Park Square, Milton Park
www.crcpress.com	Abingdon, Oxon OX 14 4RN, UK

ISBN 978-1-57808-702-0

Library of Congress Cataloging-in-Publication Data

```
Soman, A. K.
  Cloud-based solutions for healthcare it / A.K. Soman.
      p. cm.
  Includes bibliographical references and index.
  ISBN 978-1-57808-702-0 (hardcover)
1.  Medical informatics. 2.  Cloud computing.  I. Title.
  R859.7.U27S66 2011
  651.5'04261--dc22
```

                                                        2010033459

The views expressed in this book are those of the author(s) and the publisher does not assume responsibility for the authenticity of the findings/conclusions drawn by the author(s). Also no responsibility is assumed by the publishers for any damage to the property or persons as a result of operation or use of this publication and/or the information contained herein.

Printed in the United States of America

To my family

Preface

The purpose of this book is to provide an introduction to Cloud-based healthcare IT systems and to equip healthcare providers with the background necessary to evaluate and deploy Cloud-based solutions.

The American Recovery and Reinvestment Act of 2009 (ARRA) was signed into law on February 17, 2009. The Health Information Technology for Economic and Clinical Health (HITECH) provisions of ARRA include important modifications to Health Insurance Portability and Accountability Act (HIPAA). Among other things, it includes specifications pertaining to how healthcare information is to be handled by care providers.

In addition to providing guidance on effective and appropriate safeguards to be adopted, the HITECH Act makes significant financial provision for healthcare infrastructure and adoption of electronic health records (EHR) by healthcare providers. Monetary incentives are available—including to individual practices, clinics, hospitals that demonstrate "meaningful use" of EHRs.

Healthcare providers need information technology solutions that help them comply with the provisions of ARRA and also enable access to the HITECH funds earmarked for "meaningful use" of EHR. This explains the interest in evaluating 'Cloud-based' options as a means to effectively attain these twin goals.

This book covers Cloud Services in the context of Healthcare IT. In the first section, we explain what Cloud Services are, the various types of Cloud Services, the pros and cons of Cloud Services when compared to traditional in-house IT solutions, technologies that make Cloud Services possible and Cloud Service business models. In the second section, we begin by reviewing various cloud-based applications for healthcare IT. We then review the provisions of HIPAA and HITECH that pertain to Information Technology usage, and whether Cloud-based solutions can meet these provisions.

Finally we address the process of adopting Cloud solutions covering issues such as vendor evaluation, migration strategies, managing transition risks and so on. In the final section, we look at other related topics in healthcare IT, such as cloud-based Personal Health Information systems, and interoperability among healthcare IT systems. In this section we have also compiled case studies based on users of commercially available cloud solutions.

A.K. Soman
October 2010

Contents

SECTION I

INTRODUCTION TO CLOUD-BASED SYSTEMS

CHAPTER 1

What are Cloud Services?

1.1 THE TRADITIONAL IT PARADIGM

For most part during the past two decades, Information Technology vendors have either sold or licensed products to customers, who have then proceeded to treat these acquisitions as their permanent assets. For example, customers regularly bought hardware such as servers, desktops, routers, storage devices and licensed software such as Operating Systems, Productivity Applications, Practice Management Software, Billing Software, and so on. The cost of acquiring the hardware and software licenses was typically borne upfront, leaving the buyer with the subsequent responsibility of utilizing and managing these hardware and software assets.

Consider the following two examples of such acquisition and use of Information Technology assets:

Example 1:

A 2-physician family medicine practice provides basic healthcare services to a local community. In addition to the two physicians, the practice employs one administrative person ('administrator') to assist with appointments/patient scheduling and other non-clinical tasks. Each physician sees about 25 patients daily, including patients of all ages with a variety of common illnesses. Patient conditions cover a wide spectrum of health issues including chronic conditions such as hypertension, allergies, or diabetes, or just regular physicals. A typical patient encounter involves a patient calling up the clinic to fix an appointment and then arriving at the appointed time. The patient is then asked to fill out necessary forms. The administrator retrieves the patient's paper charts and records the patient's vital signs for the physician meeting. While meeting the patient, the physician reviews the charts and the vital signs, examines the patient and determines the diagnosis. Subsequently, the physician creates a treatment plan that can include medication, dietary changes, minor surgical procedure, etc. Alternatively, depending on the diagnosis, the physician may recommend more tests, refer the patient to a specialist or schedule a follow-up trip. The administrator then either completes the payment formalities with the patient or sends the reimbursement request to a billing company.

The administrator has a PC running Microsoft Windows which has Practice Management software installed on it. The Practice Management software helps with patient scheduling and appointments. It also includes a billing module that interfaces with a billing company. The practice however, does not use Electronic Health Records. It uses paper charts. The paper charts are manually filed and retrieved, and are archived in the clinic. The administrator backs up the data about patient scheduling/billing from the Practice Management system on a USB disk every day (in the form of files). Backups for one previous week are maintained in this manner. The administrator also has the same software installed on a home computer and often completes some of the work from home.

Both physicians are familiar with using computing technology. One of the physicians uses a laptop running MS Windows while the other physician uses a Macintosh Macbook. The physicians primarily use their computers to access email, and to draft and print documents, etc. The clinic has installed a local wireless network and has an internet connection which enables the physicians to access email from office. The practice has bought all of its IT assets including the computers, networking equipment, operating system software, productivity software (word processing, spreadsheets, etc.), Practice Management software, Billing software, etc. All hardware and software is upgraded periodically, usually every 2–3 years. Although the IT needs are minimal, the clinic contracts with a local firm for IT-related support on an as-required basis.

The physicians understand that their paper charts are at risk from natural disasters or incidents such as theft and fire, and hence want to transition to a system of Electronic Health Records. However they want to do so in a manner that involves minimal human and financial cost and a minimal disruption to their work.

Example 2:

As a second example, consider an accounting firm that is in the business of creating, filing and maintaining tax records for its customers. In order to deliver its services, the accounting firm provides desktop computers (e.g. Intel PCs) to it staff; each desktop computer is installed with an operating system (e.g. Microsoft Windows XP), a suite of Productivity tools (e.g. Microsoft Office) and a copy of accounting software (e.g. QuickBooks). In addition, the firm has powerful computers ('Servers') on its internal Local Area Network (LAN). One of these Servers has an attached storage device, and functions as a 'Backup Server' where all customer data and other documents are archived. Another Server hosts an email-server solution, and manages the firm's email. The accounting firm invested upfront in purchasing the computers and obtaining licenses for all the software that runs on these computers on its premises (all together referred to as its "IT infrastructure"). The accounting firm (as opposed to the vendors of hardware and software) is responsible for proper functioning of its infrastructure at all times. For this purpose the accounting firm has appointed an in-house IT professional. The accounting firm typically upgrades its hardware every couple of years and buys upgrades of various software as and when they become available. Because all assets are physically located within its premises, the accounting firm is able to enforce security policies as it feels appropriate—including restrictions on physical security, employee screening, and policies for personnel including restrictions on internet access, and so on. The firm also assumes risks such as loss of data due to theft or other natural calamity, or loss of productivity resulting from breakdown of infrastructure. It therefore pays an Insurance Company for insuring its assets such as infrastructure and data.

The accounting firm sees a non-uniform work load over the course of the year. In approximately a 2-month period prior to the dates when taxes are due, it sees extremely high workloads. These high-workload periods are also the periods when the IT infrastructure of the accounting firm is utilized to the full extent of its capacity. At other times though, the IT infrastructure is utilized to less than its full capacity. This means not all desktops are utilized, servers are running at less than the full load, and some of the licensed software is not being utilized. Figure 1.1 shows a graph of the utilization vs. capacity of the IT infrastructure around the year.

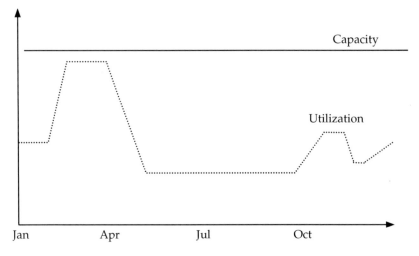

Fig. 1.1 Installed Capacity and Utilization over the year.

The periods of time when utilization is less than the capacity represent periods of inefficient usage of infrastructure i.e., periods during which the firm is unable to obtain a full return on investment made on that infrastructure. This represents a financial loss to the firm. Ideally, the accounting firm would like to see its IT infrastructure utilized to its maximum capacity around the year.

This represents a dilemma. Because the work load is not constant, the only way the accounting firm can ensure a high level of capacity utilization throughout the year is by ensuring that it's available infrastructure increases and decreases exactly in synchronization with its work load. This isn't easy to do even if the accounting firm decides to rent equipment. For one, adding and reducing rented capacity on premises is logistically difficult. Secondly, it can be fairly expensive, thereby eroding any economic gains that are sought to be achieved. Thirdly, adding resources in exact measure in which they are needed is very often not possible at all (one cannot rent 'half a server').

The two examples above demonstrate two different sets of issues with buying and maintaining IT infrastructure in-house. In the first example, the 2-physician practice wants to avoid taking on the responsibility of maintaining a full-fledged EMR/Practice Management solution in-house. In the second example, the accounting firm would like its infrastructure to scale in step with its requirements.

Cloud Services provide a potential answer to the requirements of organizations that need a fully outsourced IT solution of elastic capacity and evolving capability.

1.2 DEFINITION OF CLOUD SERVICES

The 'Cloud' represents a fundamental change to the manner in which IT services have been consumed by individuals and by organizations. This change involves a transition from "owning and managing the IT system" to "accessing IT systems as a service when required".

Cloud Services are defined as follows:

Cloud Services are Information Technology services that satisfy the following criteria:

1) *Consumers neither own the hardware on which data processing and storage happens, nor the software that performs the data processing.*
2) *Consumers have the ability to access and use the service at any time over the Internet.*

Companies that provide Cloud services are called 'Cloud Service Providers'.

Let us consider each aspect of this definition. The first part pertains to the ownership of the physical hardware and software that is used to perform data storage and data processing. Unlike in the earlier examples of the medical practice and the accounting firm where the ownership of both of these resided with them ('customer'), in the case of Cloud Services, the customer would own neither of these. The second part of the definition refers to the customer's ability to access the service remotely when it needs to use it.

The National Institute of Standards and Technology has presented a definition of Cloud-computing that can be located here [1]. Research firm IDC [2] describes Cloud-computing as "an emerging IT development, deployment and delivery model, enabling real-time delivery of products, services and solutions over the Internet." It defines Cloud Services as "Consumer and Business products, services and solutions that are delivered and consumed in real-time over the Internet". Analyst firm Gartner [3] defines it as "as a style of computing in which scalable and elastic IT-enabled capabilities are delivered as a service to external customers using Internet technologies."

The name 'Cloud Services' comes from the fact that the Internet has often pictorially been depicted as a 'Cloud'. Hence services that are accessed over the Internet are called 'Cloud Services'. Figure 1.2 is familiar to most users of Internet.

It may seem that "Cloud Services" is simply new terminology for outsourcing IT hosting to an external, third party provider. That is not accurate. There are features of Cloud offerings that differentiate them from outsourced IT hosting. We will cover these differentiators in a subsequent section. The idea of Cloud Services involves significant innovations by Service Providers both in terms of technology as well as business models. We will consider these innovations in a later chapter. Needless to say, Cloud Services are not without their drawbacks. We cover the pros and cons of Cloud Services as well.

1.3 FEATURES OF CLOUD SERVICES

In this section, we will review in detail some of the features of Cloud Services.

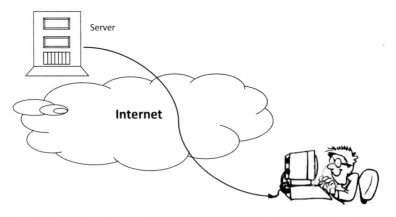

Fig. 1.2 Cloud Service Users access their IT requirements over Internet.

1.3.1 Cloud Services are accessed remotely over the Internet

Cloud Service Providers store your data and perform computations on your data at a Datacenter. [*Note: A Datacenter is a facility that houses infrastructure for secure storage and processing of data and is accessible over the internet.*] The physical location of the Datacenter could be anywhere in the world. If you need to access a Cloud service, you need to access it over a communication link, which happens to be the Internet. This also means that you can access the Cloud Service from any physical location, as long as you have an Internet connection. Datacenters are typically connected to the Internet by multiple high speed data links. The quality (data speed and link stability) of your own Internet access is hence the single most crucial element that determines the quality of user experience when accessing a Cloud Service. A reliable, fast internet connection is virtually a necessity in order to effectively utilize Cloud services.

1.3.2 Elastic Demand and Pay-As-You-Go models

You access Cloud Services '*on demand*', meaning only when you need them and utilize them only to the extent you need to. Utilization is typically measured in terms of metrics such as Data Storage space used, CPU usage, period for which you have subscribed to the service, number of concurrent user accounts you have, or any other such metric as may be appropriate for the specific Cloud Service. Cloud Service vendors build their infrastructure with the assumption that the demand for their service is likely to be '*elastic*', i.e., it could increase or decrease at any time for any of their subscribers. A particular subscriber may require a higher level of usage during a particular time (called period of high utilization) and the Cloud Service vendor's system supports periods of such high demand. The vendor bills subscribers in proportion to the subscriber's level of utilization. Periods of low utilization result in lower fees to the subscriber. Similarly, higher billings are restricted only to those durations when utilization is higher. This payment model is often referred to as a 'pay-as-you-go' model, where fees paid by the subscriber are not pre-determined, but vary as per the subscriber's level of utilization during a given period. In particular, this also means that you can subscribe to and entirely unsubscribe from a Cloud Service anytime you choose. Such a billing model significantly reduces the upfront capital investment required on part of the subscriber. On the other hand, continued usage of the Cloud Service entails a continued, recurring expense.

Some Cloud Service Providers follow a simpler billing model and charge a fixed monthly subscription fee to each of their subscribers.

1.3.3 Platform-independence

Cloud Service providers typically strive to ensure that their service can be accessed by as wide a spectrum of users as possible and build their systems appropriately. Cloud Services are usually accessible from virtually any computer with any Operating System. This includes a wide range of devices such as Windows/Apple/ Linux PCs or laptops, several types of mobile phones, handheld devices, etc. Each of these devices may be running its own operating system. The reason why such platform independence is possible is because Cloud Services are designed to be accessed through any standard Internet Browser. Virtually any combination of hardware and operating system normally supports at least one Internet Browser (e.g. Microsoft Internet Explorer, Mozilla Firefox, Opera, Safari, etc.), thereby making it possible to access the Cloud Service from virtually any system. As long as an Internet Browser (and an internet connection) is available, the Cloud Service can be accessed irrespective of the actual computing platform on which the Browser is running.

1.3.4 Shared Usage

Because different subscribers access the same Cloud-service at different times, the cloud infrastructure can be shared between different subscribers. In other words, the hardware (CPU) and the memory of a particular server may be used to perform data processing for one subscriber at a particular point in time, and the same CPU and memory may be used to perform the data processing of another subscriber at a different point in time. It is this shared usage of common resources that allows Cloud providers to offer a 'pay-as-you-go' payment model.

1.4 TYPES OF CLOUD SERVICES

There are several different types of IT requirements that can be fulfilled by Cloud Services. This section lists various classes of IT services that can be delivered from the cloud.

1.4.1 Software Cloud Services (also called SaaS i.e., Software as a Service)

These are Cloud Services wherein subscribers access and use a particular software application over Internet. These applications are also called "Web-based applications" and they run from within Internet Browsers on the user's computer. (In contrast, traditional applications that run directly on the operating system of the computer are called 'native applications'). In the case of Web-based applications, the User Interface (UI) is rendered in the Internet Browser, and the user can view or enter information through this UI. Most of the computation however is performed on the 'Servers' that reside in the Datacenter, and the user data is also stored at the Datacenter. Upgrading a Web-based application only requires the Cloud Service provider to upgrade the software resident on the servers in the Datacenter and requires no installation or intervention by the subscriber. When talking of Cloud Services in context of Healthcare IT, one is typically referring to this category of Cloud Services—the Web based applications.

Example 1: Hosted Email

A very commonly used example of a Software Cloud Service is Hosted Email (specific examples include Google Mail, Yahoo Mail, etc.). Hosted Email has been used for several years now, but earlier users of email will recollect that it was common for organizations to setup a dedicated Email server on their premises or at a Datacenter. The Email server would handle incoming and outgoing emails of the organization, store mails in mail boxes, perform email filtering, etc. Employees would use a native application on their PCs (such as Microsoft Outlook or Eudora) and this native application would communicate with the Email server of the organization to send and fetch the emails of that particular employee. The incoming/outgoing emails would then be stored physically on the user's PC. The Hosted Email solution on the other hand has the following features:

1) Hosted Email can be accessed from anywhere in the world, from any computer running any operating system; one only needs a browser to access Hosted Email.
2) All emails are stored on the storage of the Hosted Email solution provider. No data is stored on the computer which is used to access the email.
3) Users can create or discontinue their accounts at any time.

Example 2: Google Docs (Web based word processing)

Most users are familiar with Word Processing applications on PC (the most popular being Microsoft Word—bundled with MS Office). Users can buy licenses for MS Word and they subsequently own these licenses. Users can create and edit documents using MS Word. These documents are stored on the user's PC.

Google Docs [4] on the other hand, includes a 'web-based' word processor. Subscribers can create a Google Docs account over the Internet, and having done so, can access their account at any time using a computer with an Internet Browser. Creating and editing new documents is done from within the browser, and all documents thus created are stored online on data storage devices under the control of Google. Google Docs meets all the characteristics of a Software Cloud Service.

1.4.2 Computational Cloud Services (also called Cloud Computing)

This refers to a class of Cloud services that allow you to access and use computational resources (computing power, 'CPU cycles') and data storage resources over the internet. These services essentially make available a computer of customizable capacity to a subscriber who is interested in developing and running his own software programs. The following are examples of situations wherein a subscriber would need a Computational Cloud Service:

1) A situation where large amount of computational resources are required for a limited amount of time.

2) A situation where the amount of computational resources that are likely to be required is unknown upfront.

3) A situation where the amount of computational resources that are likely to be needed is highly variable over a period of time.

Effectively, this type of service makes available to the subscribers a computer that is of flexible capacity (CPU power and storage), on which subscribers can develop and run their own programs.

Example 1: Amazon's Elastic Compute Cloud (EC2) Service

Amazon's Elastic Compute Cloud (EC2) [5] is a web service that provides scalable computing capacity over the internet. Its interface allows you to obtain and configure or modify computing capacity easily at any time. EC2 claims to reduce the "time required to obtain and boot new server instances to minutes". Users can therefore add or eliminate capacity as their requirements change. Users are only billed for the capacity that they actually use. In order to use EC2, developers need to structure their applications, associated libraries and data in a standard template (called Amazon Machine Image) and upload it to Amazon's servers. Developers can then launch as many instances of these images as may be required at any time. Each of these instances needs additional computing power which is instantly made available by Amazon.

1.4.3 Cloud Web Services (also called Application Programming Interface (API) Services)

These Cloud Services encompass a class of services which allow users to access and integrate data manipulation or storage functionality (as function calls) over the Internet. Libraries of function calls are implemented by Service Providers and these can be invoked remotely by application developers from within their applications. The actual data processing or storage required to implement the functions happens on the servers of the Web Service Provider. When a function call is invoked, the function processes the data and returns the result to the application invoking the web-service. This is conceptually similar to the practice of using third party libraries while building native applications, except that in the Cloud case, the library resides on the remote servers and is accessed over the internet.

Database Web Services are a special case of Cloud Web Services. These are services where entire database capability (the database storage, as well as database operations) are performed remotely, and this remote database capability can be included as a part of your application.

Example 1: US Postal Service Web APIs

The US Postal Service [6] has published a number of web-based APIs (function calls) that can be accessed and used by application developers over the web. The Address Information API for example contains a function for ZIP Code lookup, where a correct ZIP code is returned for any address within the US. The US Postal Service maintains the database and performs the operations necessary for the ZIP Code lookup on its servers. However, anyone can access the API function from within their applications where such functionality may be required. The application calling the API can be running on any Internet connected computer, while the functions in the API run on US Postal Service's servers.

The US Postal Service has published several APIs that are available on its website.

Example 2: Intuit's QuickBase

Intuit's QuickBase [7] is an online database. The database (where the data is actually stored) is housed on Intuit's servers and is accessible over the internet. QuickBase also has an API that provides users of QuickBase the ability to access and manipulate the Quickbase data programmatically, i.e., from within their applications. All the standard database operations—creation/edits of databases, tables and records are possible via this API. Hundreds of applications leverage Intuit's QuickBase and associated API and many of those applications are themselves available as web-based applications.

1.4.4 Platform Cloud Services

These refer to a class of Cloud services that allow application developers to access and utilize a proprietary platform on the Internet for building and deploying third party applications. The platform is owned and managed by the Service Provider, who defines specifications regarding how applications may be built and deployed on the platform. Typically, Platform Cloud Services are provided by vendors who already have a large existing user base for their web services and want to offer additional applications developed by third parties to that user base. This benefits the application developers as well, who have a ready pool of prospective users to license their applications to.

Example 1: Salesforce AppExchange

Salesforce [8] offers technology solutions for various aspects of Customer Relationship Management (CRM), including sales, marketing and customer service. Force.com AppExchange is its Cloud-computing platform. Developers build applications that either extend the existing Salesforce functionality or stand-alone applications that run on Salesforce's cloud infrastructure. Such applications need to be developed in conformance to the guidelines defined by Salesforce, so that they may run on the Salesforce platform. These applications can then access data stored within the Salesforce CRM application. The AppExchange allows buyers to 'buy' (i.e., access and use) applications created by Developers on the force.com platform. There are hundreds of applications that have been developed so far on this platform.

1.5 EVOLUTION OF CLOUD SERVICES

'Cloud Services' is new terminology, but offerings based on similar ideas have existed and evolved over several decades. 'Nothing new' is often intended as a criticism of Cloud Services. For mission critical applications such as those in Healthcare however, 'nothing new' can be a plus. In this section we will review how the idea of Cloud Services has evolved over time. This background will help place Cloud Services in a historical context and provide the reader with a perspective to evaluate the services available today.

1.5.1 Examples of early Cloud Services

Service Bureaus, Mainframes and ASPs are three prominent examples of what can be called precursors to Cloud Services of today.

1.5.1.1 *Service Bureaus*

The earliest manifestation of the idea of "Cloud Services" was the Service Bureau of 1960s. A Service Bureau was any company that provided a combination of technology, infrastructure and human services to customers on an as-required basis. Service Bureau Corporation (SBC) was a subsidiary of IBM (later sold to Control Data Corporation) that specialized in providing services that were very similar to Cloud services of today. Customers (typically financial institutions) could upload, store and process data on SBC's computers remotely on a time sharing basis.

American Data Services founded in 1956 was another Cloud Provider that provided commercial and bank data processing services. It advertised itself as follows [9] "[Amerian Data Services is] *a computer service company that deals exclusively with financial institutions, we offer up-to-date computing facilities and applications software that independent banks can use to compete in this changing arena. Just as important, our data communications network that links each bank with our central data processing facility is so sophisticated that it's as if each bank had its own inhouse computer system.*"

Several decades ago, Service Bureaus offered Cloud-based Services for exactly the same business reasons that Cloud providers offer them today. These business reasons included desire on part of customers to avoid investment in expensive hardware that would be idle for most of the time. Customers much rather preferred to access a powerful computing platform whenever they needed it. Interestingly, network stability and security were key issues for customers even at that time.

1.5.1.2 Mainframes

Mainframes are computers with very large processing and storage capacity and are called thus because all processing units and communication buses are housed within a single cabinet or frame. Mainframes have been used for a long time by universities that need to make computing facilities available to their campus communities. Consoles are used to connect to the mainframes over communication links. The applications run on the Mainframe and data storage happens centrally as well. Commands entered over the console are communicated to the Mainframe, and the results are communicated back for viewing on the console. Students are often metered for their usage similar to the manner in which Cloud Services are metered today.

1.5.1.3 Application Service Providers (ASPs)

Application Service Providers (ASP) were businesses in the 1990s that managed and offered the use of software on an "as required basis" to customers over a network. Independent Software Vendors licensed software to the ASPs who then installed the software on their own computers in a Datacenter. ASPs then provided access to the software to the end users over a network (typically the Internet). The consumer usually used a 'thin client', i.e., a small piece of software running on the consumer's computer in order to access the software running on the ASP's computers in the Datacenter.

The primary benefits to the consumer were the fact that the consumer did not have to invest in expensive hardware and software upfront, did not have to hire and train an in-house IT team, and did not have to worry about the maintenance or upgrades to the software. Any software that was complex and expensive therefore became an ideal choice for support through the ASP model. This is the reason why many ASPs got into the business of supporting complex software such as ERP systems, financial systems, etc. ASPs billed either on per user basis or on a monthly basis, much like the Cloud service providers of today.

The ASP business model unfortunately did not succeed, and a vast majority of the companies that got into the ASP business perished. There were several reasons for this. Firstly, the ASPs had to invest in the cost of commissioning the entire infrastructure upfront, including setting up servers, commissioning high capacity communication lines, purchasing software from ISVs, employing and training staff, etc., whereas the revenues came in only over a period of time. Many ASPs underestimated the upfront cost, and it was not easy making money from monthly payments from customers. Secondly, ASPs stayed away from offering customization services. This meant that the customer was left without recourse, if he needed customization or associated services.

Cloud Service providers have an identical value proposition to what the ASPs did, but several factors have changed since then, creating optimism that today's Cloud Providers will not meet the same fate that befell the ASPs. Firstly, the cost of infrastructure has significantly reduced since the 1990s. The Cloud service providers of today incur much smaller infrastructure costs upfront when compared to ASPs in the 1990s. Secondly, ASPs did not offer any substantial improvement in the feature set, quality, or usability of software—they were only setting up software developed by ISVs (Independent Software Vendors) to be used by final consumers. On the other hand, Cloud Providers today play the role of ISVs as well as ASPs. They own the software running on their servers and are in a position to evolve their offerings in sync with the needs of the consumers.

1.5.2 Cloud Service Adoption and Key Cloud Drivers

Across several industry verticals, vendors offer Cloud-based solutions that compete with the on-site systems sold by traditional providers. As per a survey conducted by Mimecast in October 2009 [10] of IT users across industries, 36% of respondents were using Cloud-based solutions compared to 64% who were not. Even more important, 70% of those who were using Cloud-based solutions said they would move additional applications to the cloud. These numbers were fairly constant across various industry verticals including Healthcare. An IDC Survey conducted earlier [11] showed consistent results. It showed a slightly lesser number of respondents already using Cloud-based services at that time, with a third of all respondents indicating a desire to enhance the level of Cloud usage in the next 3 years. Cost and 'agility' (the ability to get started quickly) were seen as the primary reasons for moving to Cloud-based applications in both the Mimecast Survey, as well as the IDC survey. Another point worth noting from the Mimecast Survey is that the most commonly used Cloud-based applications were Email, Data Storage and archiving. ERP and Sales Management systems were least likely to have been moved to the Cloud.

The above data indicates two things. Firstly, the idea of Cloud-based services is gaining rapid acceptance among users of IT systems. Secondly, adoption is led by a certain category of applications while adoption is lower for other categories of applications that are more complex.

Many large established ISVs (Independent Software Vendors) who have traditionally offered on-premise software now also provide Cloud-based systems. For example, Microsoft has launched its Windows Azure platform [12] which offers "a flexible, familiar environment for developers to create cloud applications and services". SQL Azure is a fully relational Cloud database solution. Amazon EC2 as we have seen earlier is a flexible Cloud-based computing platform, and Amazon S3 is a Cloud-based relational database. Similarly, IBM offers "Smart Business solutions" for application development, test and storage on its cloud platform [13]. There are literally thousands of other vendors who now provide Cloud-based solutions for various industry verticals.

The following are some of the 'key cloud drivers'—i.e., factors responsible for the momentum towards adoption of Cloud-based solutions.

1.5.2.1 Mobility and Mobile computing

Today's workforce is increasingly mobile, and for many people, a hand-held device is the most preferred means to access data. It is estimated that at this time, there are 2 Billion mobile phones in use around the world, and at least 30% of them are data capable. The number of data capable mobiles is growing rapidly. It is therefore preferable that any organization's information be accessible from mobile devices, from anywhere, for the benefit of the mobile workforce of the organization. Globally accessible data is best stored in the cloud as opposed to within an organization. Mobile computing is hence one of the key drivers towards Cloud-based applications and Cloud-based data storage.

1.5.2.2 The role of Social Networks

Changing human attitudes and customer conditioning has a huge role to play in the acceptance of a particular technology or offering. The phenomena of social networks and their global reach, particularly among younger audience has played a significant role in making Cloud services more acceptable today. Most users of social networking sites are perfectly comfortable uploading their personal photos and information to third party social network providers such as Facebook, Myspace and others. When these individuals are confronted with a potential choice of hosting their business data or work-related materials with a 'Cloud provider', they are much more likely to be willing to do so.

1.5.2.3 Economics

While IT budgets may not necessarily shrink in terms of the amounts, CIOs and consumers of IT now expect to get far more for their dollar than they did earlier—and sooner. Furthermore, there is little patience for solutions that take months to install or implement. Cloud Services fit the bill perfectly on both counts. Cloud services allow users to treat IT as an operational expense rather than as a capital expense.

1.5.2.4 Vendor Preference

One of the strongest forces driving adoption of Cloud services may well be the cloud vendors themselves. It is a lot easier and cheaper to offer a new product as a Cloud Service rather than as packaged software. Cloud-based offerings are also significantly easier to distribute, and easier to maintain and support as well. Therefore, most emerging companies or 'startups' (who are most likely to offer novel and innovative solutions) prefer to offer their products in the form of Cloud Services. Cloud Service providers are an ecosystem. One provider of Cloud Services often uses Cloud Services from another provider as a part of his solutions. Taking the cue from smaller companies, larger, more established ISVs are doing this too. We already looked at the example of Microsoft, which after years of having dominated the packaged software market on the PC platform, is now introducing several products as Cloud Services.

1.5.3 The future

With the momentum they now have, it is possible that Cloud-based offerings may well become the preferred mechanism to deliver and consume Information Technology across most industries in the future. Many analysts and industry leaders believe that the future of Computing is in the Cloud [14]–[17]. The Internet Browser shall take place of operating systems in the future, and all data of all individuals will be stored in the Cloud, always accessible from anywhere. This data will be seamlessly shared across all applications that need the data. The broad popularity of Cloud-based social networks only indicates the wide-spread acceptance of the cloud delivery model among Internet users. Some [18] believe that computing will be like a utility, available on demand much like electricity is. Merrill Lynch projects Cloud-computing revenues will reach $160 billion in 2011.

IDC estimates the Cloud-computing market will reach $42 billion in 2012 [19].

Healthcare however, is very different from most other verticals. Firstly, the industry is extensively regulated and any solution needs to comply with these regulations. Secondly, there is significantly higher sensitivity of data involved when compared to other verticals. There are penalties for not having strong data privacy and security safeguards in place. Thirdly, there are many different entities within the healthcare industry that need to interact and exchange data with each other.

On the other hand, Cloud-based systems are considered by many to be the easiest to use when it comes to Electronic Health Records. Cloud-based systems have recently certainly gained recognition within the Healthcare Industry. Nothing demonstrates this more than the fact that the Department of Health and Human Services is looking to deploy Cloud-based customer relationship and project management software for its Regional Extension Centers [20]. The software will help the Regional Extension Centers to more effectively track and manage medical providers implementing electronic health record (EHR) systems. The Cloud-computing CRM and project management technology for this project comes from salesforce.com

REFERENCES

[1] http://csrc.nist.gov/groups/SNS/Cloud-computing/index.html

[2] http://blogs.idc.com/ie/?p=190

[3] http://www.gartner.com/it/page.jsp?id=1035013

[4] http://docs.google.com

[5] http://aws.amazon.com/ec2/

[6] http://www.usps.com/webtools/

[7] http://quickbase.intuit.com

[8] http://www.salesforce.com

[9] http://findarticles.com/p/articles/mi_m0CMN/is_n1_v22/ai_601498/

[10] http://www.mimecast.com/cloudsurvey

[11] http://blogs.idc.com/ie/?p=730

[12] http://www.microsoft.com/windowsazure/

[13] http://www.ibm.com/ibm/cloud/

[14] http://pewresearch.org/pubs/1623/future-Cloud-computing-technology-experts

[15] http://www.readwriteweb.com/archives/why_cloud_computing_is_the_future_of_mobile.php

[16] http://stevenbutler.com/2009/10/11/cloud-os/

[17] http://research.microsoft.com/en-us/news/features/ccf-022409.aspx

[18] The Big Switch: Rewiring the World, from Edison to Google, Nicholas Carr, W. W. Norton & Company, 2008

[19] http://www.von.com/articles/2008/12/Cloud-computing-part-2-gauging-the-opportunity.aspx

[20] http://gcn.com/articles/2010/02/19/health-and-human-services-Cloud-computing.aspx

CHAPTER 2

Benefits and Drawbacks of Cloud Services

In the previous chapter, we covered the definition of Cloud services and the different types of Cloud services. We also reviewed examples of previous manifestations of similar ideas.

Various surveys including those by IDC [1], Gartner [2], Mimecast [3] and others indicate a large and rapidly growing market for Cloud services across various industries. These adoption numbers seem to indicate two things: firstly, that Cloud-based services have certain advantages over the traditional packaged software and secondly, that some percentage of prospective users continue to have reservations about using Cloud services.

Several of the perceived advantages/drawbacks of Cloud services are industry specific. Issues that are relevant in one industry vertical may not be seen as important in another industry. In this chapter we shall review the advantages and disadvantages of Cloud services in the context of the healthcare industry.

The HITECH Act provides financial incentives for adoption of Electronic Medical Records (EMR) by all healthcare providers including office physician practices and clinics. Numerous physician practices are therefore in the process of evaluating EMR systems and identifying one that best meets their needs in addition to meeting the regulatory requirements. There are broadly two classes of EMR solutions to choose from: a) the in-house solutions that have traditionally been used and b) the more recent Cloud-based solutions.

Evaluation of IT solutions is typically performed on the basis of criteria such as functionality, ease of use, total cost associated with using the solution, ability to comply with regulations, and so on. In this chapter, we will look at the merits and demerits of each approach (in-house vs. cloud) in the context of such evaluation criteria.

Not all companies manage their in-house IT infrastructure with equal efficiency and not every Cloud Service offers similar functionality. In this chapter we will focus on the inherent merits/demerits of the two approaches rather than reviewing and comparing any specific solutions.

The key criteria for evaluating IT solutions are discussed below:

2.1 FUNCTIONALITY AND EASE OF USE

The overall functionality of a product and its ease of use are probably the first criteria that a buyer looks for in any IT product. 'Functionality' covers the feature set of the system, i.e., the various different operations that system can perform—the things that the system can do. For example, evaluating the functionality of the system involves asking questions such as:

1) Does the system allow the entry of all data that needs to be captured?
2) Does the system produce all the charts and reports that the physician or nurse may want to view?
3) Does the system provide the ability to send out easily all the billing related communications and track collections?
4) Does the system provide suitable linkages between various aspects of the practice such as between the EMR module and the practice management module, ePrescription module, Billing module, and so on?

Medical Practitioners need to create a-priori a checklist of capabilities (functions) they need in a system they procure. This list should be broken into two parts—one part comprising items that are essential and second part comprising items that are good to have.

'Ease of use', as the name suggests pertains to how easy it is to use the overall system and exercise its functionality. While 'ease-of-use' is a subjective criterion, users typically seek to quantify it by asking questions such as:

1) Is all necessary information available on each screen as it should be?
2) Are the screens cluttered with too much information which makes it hard to find the specific information one is looking for?
3) Does the same data have to be entered more than once?
4) How many 'mouse clicks' does it take to perform the most common operations?
5) Is it possible to customize the workflows?
6) Is there more than one way to do each of the most common operations?
7) Does the system have validations for common data fields which notify the user of typos?
8) Is the system forgiving of genuine human errors? That is, in case of genuine human error, is it possible to quickly roll back or does one need to start over again?
9) Does the system support all the templates that your specialty needs?

When it comes to healthcare IT, there are very few things that a native application (in-house system) can do which a Cloud-based service cannot. Today's web-technologies make it possible for a Cloud-based service to provide virtually all the functionality that a Healthcare provider would seek in an IT system. It is also possible to create Cloud-based systems that are easy to use and support the different workflows that healthcare providers require. This applies to all specialties.

There is an impression that Cloud-based systems work slower than in-house products due to the fact that data communication happens over internet connections. While this is theoretically true—in the case of Cloud services data travels over multiple hubs on the internet and there is latency—in practice, this difference is marginal if one uses a high speed connection with low latency.

From a standpoint of functionality and ease of use therefore, both in-house systems and Cloud-based systems can be considered on-par. There is virtually nothing that makes an in-house system intrinsically better than a Cloud-based system from a functionality standpoint or vice versa.

Note: One area where in-house systems can potentially provide superior functionality is when an IT system has to be directly interfaced with other data collection devices such as glucometers, blood-pressure monitors, etc which directly enter the readings into the system. Even in this case, it is possible for Cloud-based systems to provide this functionality with 'plug-ins', i.e., small modules that run natively within the browser.

2.2 COST

Several independent surveys of physician practices have revealed that high costs are a significant barrier that prevents a wider adoption of EMR. For example, a study [4], "Electronic Health Records in Ambulatory Care—A National Survey of Physicians," was published in June 2008 in an article by the *New England Journal of Medicine*. It said that 66% of the respondents who did not have EMR cited 'costs' as the main obstacle. In another study of 5000 family physicians [5], more than 60% cited affordability as the top barrier for EHR adoption.

The cost of buying and installing an in-house EMR system (including the hardware, software, training, etc.) for a small clinic can be around US $10,000 or even higher, depending on the size of the practice. Added to this initial cost are the recurring maintenance costs. Office Physicians and smaller clinics may find this a significant investment to make. Proponents of Cloud Services claim that Cloud Services can deliver EMR capability at a significantly lower cost vis-à-vis licensed in-house software, and hence Cloud Services are the way to accelerate EMR adoption.

When a Medical practice calculates the 'cost' of a particular solution, it really needs to determine the "total cost of adoption" of a particular solution—whether the solution is in-house or Cloud-based. This "total cost of adoption" includes not just the cost of licensing software or the subscription fees, but includes every investment of time, resources and money that goes towards utilization of that solution on an on-going basis. Not all costs can be easily quantified. Nevertheless they need to be estimated and factored into the equation.

The "total cost of adoption" can be classified under two heads —The "one-time costs" and the "recurring costs". In this section we will discuss the different cost-items that can be listed under each of the two heads.

2.2.1 Initial Infrastructure costs (One time)

One-time costs are typically borne upfront—at the outset—before a solution is usable.

In the case of in-house IT systems, one-time costs include costs of:

1) Hardware
   a. computers for staff
   b. servers for running the software
   c. printers
   d. networking devices such as routers, modems, data storage devices
   e. storage devices for data backups
   f. hand-held or mobile devices if applicable

2) Software
   a. operating systems for staff computers and servers
   b. general software such as productivity software, etc not directly connected with healthcare.
   c. Healthcare software including EMR, Practice Management, ePrescription, Billing software, etc. that is sought to be deployed and used.
   d. Security software to protect against cyber-attacks.

3) Physical Infrastructure
   a. secured & controlled space and racks to house your servers and networking equipment,
   b. additional air-conditioning/clean room installation,
   c. additional electrical backup systems including batteries, generators to ensure continuous supply.
   d. Internet connectivity to ensure patient information is available to patients via 'patient portals'.

In the case of Cloud services, the one-time costs include:

1) Hardware
   a. computers for staff
   b. printers
   c. networking devices such as routers, modems, data storage devices
   d. hand-held or mobile devices if applicable

2) Software
   a. operating systems for staff computers
   b. other software such as productivity software, etc. not directly connected with healthcare.
   c. Security software to protect against cyber-attacks.

3) Physical Infrastructure
   a. Internet connectivity to ensure access to the Cloud service.

Comparison: When utilizing Cloud-based services, a practice saves significant upfront costs because it does not have to put in place additional infrastructure to support the in-house IT setup and it does not need to invest in buying servers or software upfront. Secondly, while using Cloud-based solutions, staff computers can be less sophisticated because they are used to only access the Cloud service and not to perform actual computation or storage. With in-house systems, one needs to provision for back-up and failover, as well.

From a point of view of upfront infrastructure cost (capital investment), Cloud-based services are substantially more attractive than the in-house option.

2.2.2 On-going Infrastructure costs (Recurring)

These are the costs the practice will incur periodically (i.e., either monthly/yearly/quarterly or simply from time-to-time) in order to ensure continuous availability and use of the IT solution.

In the case of in-house IT, this includes:

1) Real Estate (typically, rent associated with the additional space taken up by servers and supporting infrastructure)
2) Higher Utility bills resulting from the additional infrastructure

3) Maintenance cost of the additional infrastructure

4) Cost of trained personnel to maintain and manage the IT infrastructure

5) Periodic upgrades to software/hardware from time to time

6) Cost of Insurance for your IT infrastructure and also the data

In the case of Cloud Services, the on-going costs include:

1) Cost of subscribing to the service. One needs to pay the Cloud Service vendor periodically for using the Cloud Service(s) being provided. Different vendors follow different subscription models—but usually, the subscription fees are directly proportional to the level of utilization. Utilization itself is measured in terms of one or more parameters such as the number and/or type of users, duration of use, amount of storage required, and so on. Examples of Cloud service billing models are:

Example 1: Per-user-per-month or Per-user-per-year

In this model, the Cloud provider bills based on the number of distinct user accounts that you need for your practice. It is possible that physician accounts are charged differently from nurse accounts (if the software supports such a differentiation). Billing is either per month or per year (typically yearly billing comes with a discount to the monthly rate).

Example 2: Per records

In this model, the Cloud provider bills you on the basis of your actual consumption of specific resources—for example, the number of patients whose records you actually store, or the storage space in Gigabytes you utilize, etc.

2) Cost resulting from higher Internet usage. Because the internet connection is the single most important point of failure in the context of Cloud services, having high speed internet connections with full redundancy is necessary. Full redundancy refers to having a minimum of two different internet connections from two different vendors based on two different technologies (for e.g. one wired cable connection and another a WiMax connection). High speed Internet connections typically require a higher monthly subscription fee.

3) Cost of personnel to manage technology and relationship with the Cloud Service provider. Unlike the case of in-house systems, utilizing Cloud-based systems does not require dedicated personnel. However, someone within the practice does need to periodically spend time working with the Cloud provider for issues such as seeking support when needed, managing user accounts, reviewing audit data, generating compliance documentation, upgrading browsers with security patches and even occasionally backing up data. In other words, although the personnel costs are much lower, they are not zero.

Comparison: A comparison of recurring infrastructure related costs depends on the specific numbers associated with the cost items listed above. These could vary based on Cloud service provider, infrastructure vendor, etc.

2.2.3 Migration Cost, Risk and Productivity Loss (One-time)

If a practice is moving from one type of a system to another (such as from an in-house system to a Cloud-based system or from a paper-based system to an EMR), it involves a 'migration cost'—which is the price that the practice would pay in terms of lost productivity in the interim, the price of potentially maintaining two types of systems for a limited amount of time, and so on. Some of these costs are hard to quantify, but are costs nevertheless.

The process of migrating to a new solution is typically preceded by a period in which the practice must consider all the options and make a selection from among those available. This involves researching several solutions and determining one best suited to the needs of the practice. This can be a time consuming process, requiring the time and attention of several individuals within a practice. Selecting a solution requires review of available literature, and it could even involve using each solution for a limited amount of time. Legal agreements such as User agreements and Service Level Agreements have to be carefully reviewed in order to understand liabilities, obligations and legal recourse.

Once a particular solution is selected, the practice needs to transition from its existing workflows to the new workflows. This holds true whether one is beginning with a new EMR solution, i.e., using an EMR for the first time or whether one is migrating from an on-premise solution to a Cloud-based solution. Such migration takes time, and unless done meticulously is often prone to accidents —data being lost or being incorrectly formatted, information being overlooked or wrongly entered, processes being incorrectly mapped, passwords being lost or compromised and so on.

Such a migration entails loss of productivity because staff has to undergo training, and settling into a new process naturally takes some time. During the course of the transition, most practices see a significant drop in the number of patients they can see daily.

Cloud-based solutions are easier to evaluate or try. They require no significant investment in terms of hardware or software. Most Cloud service providers provide prospective customers with a 'free trial period' during which potential subscribers may experiment with the service and verify that it meets their requirements. The potential subscriber may then make a decision based on the experience with using the service during the free trial period. Migration risks can be substantially reduced by availing the free trail periods provided by most cloud vendors. Such a free trial period is typically not available with in-house solutions. Migration risks with in-house solutions are therefore higher.

Comparison: Cloud-based solutions require virtually no investment if a practice wants to tryout the solutions for limited time. The migration risks for a Cloud-based solution are typically lower. The cost of personnel training, and the productivity loss is an equal factor in both cases.

2.2.4 Cost of Compliance

HIPAA and HITECH impose considerable responsibility on part of providers in terms of ensuring compliance with their provisions. This includes performing risk assessments, conducting audits, generating documentation, reporting compliance with various aspects of meaningful use requirements, and so on. These costs are likely to be identical in case of on-site systems and Cloud-based systems especially if the practice works with external consultants.

We will cover compliance aspects in a subsequent chapter.

2.2.5 Cost Comparison Summary

Users of Cloud services incur on-going expenses rather than significant upfront capital expenses. While a numerical comparison of the 'total cost of ownership' would depend on specific vendor pricing, it is generally likely that the total cost of ownership is lesser for Cloud-based solutions when compared to in-house solutions.

2.3 SECURITY

HIPAA includes a 'Privacy Rule' and a 'Security Rule' which together provide guidelines for protecting the electronic health data of patients. There are penalties for non-compliance with either rule. Healthcare providers therefore need to ensure that the solution and systems they put in place comply with the requirements of these rules.

Healthcare information is sensitive personal information, and unauthorized access to healthcare information is a breach of a person's privacy. By their very definition, Cloud Services store and process your data on infrastructure that physically resides outside your premises, and therefore outside of your control. Your data is transferred over the public Internet, between your office and the Provider's Datacentre. Furthermore, the convenience of 'anytime, anywhere access' means that your data can become accessible to anyone from any location who happens to get hold of your password.

The IDC survey as well as the Mimecast survey referred to earlier both indicate that *"Security"* is the foremost concern for people planning to use Cloud-based solutions.

Security has as much to do with people and processes in an organization as it does with the actual technology involved. The underlying technology is only one component from among several that determine the overall security provided by a system. Secondly, there are tradeoffs involved in every system—between ease of use and convenience on one hand and security on the other. In this section, we will review Cloud-based systems and in-house systems from a security perspective.

2.3.1 What is 'Data Security'?

Before we examine Cloud-based or in-house systems, we need to define 'security' in the context of healthcare data. Data is inherently different from physical goods whose 'security' we are familiar with. Physical goods are usually secured by keeping them under lock and key or under surveillance. Data is different however, and 'Data Security' has three different aspects:

2.3.1.1 Confidentiality

Confidentiality of data refers to the requirement that no person who is not authorized by the owner of the data should be able to access the data ('access' the data means either read or copy or utilize it in any other way). Confidentiality of data is said to be violated if the data is accessed by anyone who should not have access to it. A user of a Cloud service needs the guarantee that the confidentiality of data is maintained while the data is in transit to and from the Cloud provider, and while it resides within the infrastructure of the Cloud provider. This means that no one should be able to make use of the data while it is in transit or while it resides on the infrastructure of the Cloud provider.

Data is stored as a sequence of bits in any IT system (often called the 'bit stream'). Confidentiality is usually guaranteed by *encrypting* the data. Encryption is a reversible process that renders the data unreadable and unusable. It converts the original data bit-stream into another data bit-stream called the encrypted data. Encrypted data does not resemble the original data and the information contained in the original data is virtually impossible to obtain from the encrypted data. The process of encryption is performed based on a secret character string called a 'key'—use of different key during encryption results in a different stream of encrypted data. Encrypted data can be converted back to the original data ('decrypted') using a decryption key, which is either the same as the encryption key or mathematically related to it (this depends on the specific algorithm used to encrypt the data). Encrypted data is not compromised even if it is accessed by an unauthorized person, unless the person also has access to the decryption key. That means, someone with access to the encrypted data does not have access to the original data unless he also has the decryption key.

Confidentiality is maintained as long as:

1) Data is stored in an encrypted fashion, *and*
2) Decryption key is kept confidential,

Further information on data encryption can be found in [6] [7].

2.3.1.2 *Integrity*

Integrity of data refers to the requirement that data not be corrupted and not be modified without the explicit knowledge of its owner. A user of a Cloud service needs the assurance at all times that his data stored with the Cloud provider is not modified or altered in any way either by an inadvertent error or by malice. Similarly, the Cloud-service user needs the assurance that his data in transit from the data center to his computer is not modified in any manner or corrupted.

Integrity of data (whether in transit or in storage) is guaranteed by incorporating a cryptographic hash. The cryptographic hash is a code word that is generated from the original data. If a change is made to the data (howsoever minor), the cryptographic hash of the modified data will also be different.

To ensure Integrity, cryptographic hash of the data is computed and securely stored/communicated. When the data is to be used, its cryptographic hash is recomputed and compared with the original cryptographic hash to ensure that the data has not changed. More information on cryptographic hash can be found in [6] [7].

2.3.1.3 *Availability*

Availability of data refers to the requirement that the user's data is available at any time the user desires to access or use it. Unavailability of data may be temporary (as in a situation wherein the IT systems are being upgraded), or it can be permanent. Permanent loss of data is a catastrophic situation, and it is the responsibility of those managing the IT Infrastructure (either the in-house administrator or the Cloud service provider as the case may be) to put in place systems and infrastructure that guard against such data loss.

Availability is typically guaranteed by ensuring remote backup of all data, ensuring redundancy of data communication (bandwidth), and proper and safe storage of all encryption keys.

Any situation that leads to either loss of confidentiality, breach of integrity or non-availability of user data is a security failure in the context of Cloud services.

We will now review the points of security vulnerability for in-house systems and Cloud-based systems.

2.3.2 Points of Vulnerability in an In-house IT System

Figure 2.1 shows the different elements of an in-house IT framework.

The computers within the practice are connected via a local area network (LAN). The network could be either a wired (Ethernet) network or a wireless network. The primary installation of the software is on the Application server; data is stored in a storage server and backed up periodically on storage devices. The software on the server is accessed by the individual computers used by clinical and non-clinical staff.

1) The individual computers are vulnerable to corruption with viruses and other malware. Viruses and malware is usually communicated via infected media (USB/disks), infected email or by visiting compromised websites. However, by installing commercially available security software on these computers or a network based security software, this vulnerability can be addressed. It is necessary to enforce a rule that prevents media (USB, disks, etc.) from being taken in or out of the practice.

2) If the LAN is not connected to the Internet, it minimizes the scope for malware infecting these computers. However, the requirement of patient portals and interoperability make it necessary that there be an external network connection. The external network connection represents vulnerability. This vulnerability can also be addressed by commercial security products such as firewalls.

3) The contractors/consultants/employees working with the system represent the third point of vulnerability. The practice needs to ensure that anyone who deals with the IT systems and health information is screened for background, and access is provided only on a need to know basis. The practice needs to install physical access controls and surveillance equipment to monitor the premises for unauthorized access.

4) The premises are susceptible to risks from natural or other disasters—floods, earthquake, theft, fire etc putting at risk the data stored within the office. The practice can counter this risk by frequently backing up all data to an offsite location.

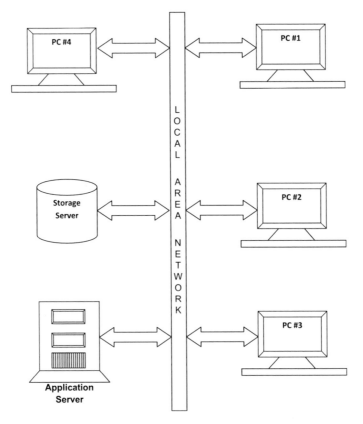

Fig. 2.1 Inhouse IT Network.

2.3.3 Points of Vulnerability in a Cloud Services Framework

Figure 2.2 shows the different elements of the IT infrastructure in a Cloud services framework.

We will now examine the points of vulnerability when it comes to using a Cloud-based service.

2.3.3.1 Individual Computers used to access the Cloud service

The computer that is used to access the Cloud service is the first element in a chain of devices involved in the consumption of Cloud services. This computer is internet-connected via a LAN and could be infected with malware such as, viruses, worms, keystroke recording agents, etc unless it is properly secured.

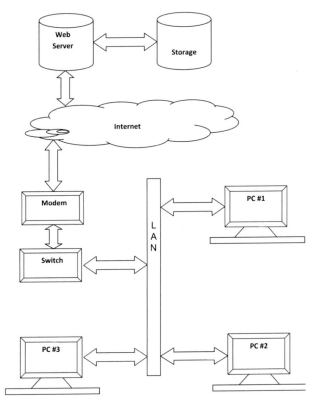

Fig. 2.2 Accessing a Cloud Service.

One of the key benefits of Cloud Services is the fact that they can be accessed from any internet connected computer and at any time. That means a user does not have to be within the office premises in order to access the Cloud service. Accessing the Cloud Service from a computer outside your office that is potentially infected presents another security risk. For example, consider a situation where an employee of your practice accesses the Cloud service from an infected home computer or from a cyber café. Suppose the employee's password is recorded and transmitted using a keystroke logging malware on the infected computer. The password can then be subsequently used to access the healthcare information stored in the cloud.

Use of Cloud Services also magnifies the damage that a disgruntled employee or contractor can do. It is much easier for such an individual to download and misuse data from a location outside your practice, without having to go through the physical controls that are enforced within your office. Such risks are lower when using in-house IT because of the presence of a number of physical access controls and security systems that flag the copying or downloading of data.

While using Cloud services the following precautions need to be taken:

1) Healthcare practices need to ensure that all employees access the service only from computers that are guaranteed to be free of viruses or other malware. Healthcare practices can take steps to ensure that computers within their premises are always clean from malware, but it is harder to ensure that computers in employee's homes are also similarly clean because it requires meticulous compliance on part of the employee.

2) Healthcare practices need to be careful about managing employee transitions. Cloud Service access needs to be immediately disabled for departed employees, disgruntled employees/contractors, and those who you can no longer trust with data.

To summarize, ubiquitous access to Cloud services is both a benefit as well as a drawback. The fact that Cloud services can be accessed from any computer at any time creates risk that is not present for in-house IT systems. There are ways in which these risks can be mitigated, particularly by the Cloud Provider, as we will see in a later chapter.

2.3.3.2 *The Internet Browser*

Most Cloud Services are accessed through a standard Internet browser. This is certainly a convenience, but it also has security implications. Firstly, any security flaw within the browser impacts the security of your healthcare data. While standard browsers (such as Microsoft's Internet Explorer or Mozialla's Firefox) are stable, occasional security flaws have been reported in both of them [8] [9], particularly after a new version is released. It is important to immediately upgrade your browsers whenever security patches are released.

The second potential issue with running services in a browser is the fact that the same browser is also used by employees to visit other websites. Browsers have 'security settings' and it is possible that employees forget to change their browser security settings when they visit a different site. This can potentially result in a situation where an employee sets a lower security setting in order to run an authentic Cloud service from your trusted vendor, but then forgets to set the security setting to a higher level while he browses another potentially dangerous site. This risk is eliminated by ensuring that the computers within the practice are used only to access genuine work-related websites and no other websites. This is easy to do with commercially available tools.

2.3.3.3 The communication channel

While accessing a Cloud service, data is communicated both ways—from user computer to the Datacenter (where the Cloud Service Provider's infrastructure is housed) and back over Internet. The Internet is a public medium, and normally, data carried over this medium is susceptible to eavesdropping and interference unless it is encrypted and secured.

Therefore, Cloud services secure the data in transit (between your computer and provider's servers) using standard data security protocols such as HTTPS (Hypertext Transfer Protocol—Secure). When you access the Cloud provider site using your Browser, the remote site authenticates itself to the Browser with a certificate issued by a trusted authority. This essentially tells the Browser that it is now talking with the genuine Cloud Provider site and not with another site. The process of authentication is followed by exchange of 'keys' to encrypt/decrypt all data that is transferred over the internet in both directions. The HTTPS protocol ensures the confidentiality and integrity of all data in transit between the user's computer and the Cloud Provider's infrastructure. More information on the HTTPS protocol is available in [10].

Some Cloud services use HTTPS only to communicate user passwords. This isn't good enough. The Cloud service provider must use HTTPS for all data transfers.

2.3.3.4 *Cloud Service Provider Infrastructure*

There are several points of potential security failure within the Cloud Service provider's infrastructure. Managing them is entirely the responsibility of the Service provider, and a consumer can do little in terms of minimizing the security risks within that infrastructure. Nevertheless, it is worthwhile to understand what those security risks are, since they help the consumer ask the right questions while evaluating various Cloud-based offerings.

The security challenges within the Cloud Provider's operation include protecting the IT systems against cyber attacks, ensuring physical safety of the infrastructure, implementing procedures for data backup & recovery, creating and implementing internal processes and policies for personnel, etc.

2.3.3.4.1 *Cyber attacks against server infrastructure*

Any server infrastructure that is accessible over the internet is vulnerable to cyber attacks. These include: Denial of Service Attacks—relying on large number of simultaneous requests hitting the servers so that the servers either fail entirely or are unable to process genuine requests; Database injection attacks which attempt to inject malicious queries into the system database via text fields; or other attacks that seek to exploit system vulnerabilities in order to get malicious code to execute on the servers. The Cloud Service provider needs to implement security tools that fortify his IT infrastructure against cyber-attacks over the internet. This includes blocking traffic on all except authorized ports, implementing firewalls that filter incoming data on open ports, detecting malware in incoming data, antivirus software that continually runs on the servers, and so on.

Web Infrastructure security is in itself an established industry, and there are many commercially available security applications and tools that can protect the Cloud Provider's infrastructure from the threats mentioned above.

2.3.3.4.2 *Physical Security*

Cloud Infrastructure is housed in Datacenters. The Datacenters are vulnerable to many types of physical risks just as the IT infrastructure within the premises of your practice is vulnerable to physical risks. As mentioned earlier, this includes disasters such as fire, earthquakes, storms, floods, as well as risks of human intrusion, theft, and so on.

There are several standards from industry bodies that define guidelines for setting up and operating Datacenters and most modern Datacenters comply with these guidelines. Datacenters not only have access to latest security technologies, processes and systems but also have the means to adopt them. It is probably true that data inside Datacenters is likely to be better protected than data within your premises.

2.3.3.4.3 Data Storage Security

Cloud Service Providers store a large amount of data from a large number of subscribers in their databases housed within Datacenters. These databases are indirectly accessible over the Internet and therefore need to be secured. Hackers usually prefer to hack into systems that hold millions of records (Cloud service provider) than go after systems that hold a few thousand records (your practice). When you utilize a Cloud Service, your data is now among those millions of records with the Cloud service provider. The Provider therefore needs to implement a much higher level of security than a typical physician practice and prevent unauthorized access to their database.

Cloud Service Providers have a genuine need to store the passwords of their users. For example genuine users sometimes accidentally lose or forget their passwords. It is contingent upon the Provider to make the password available to such a user. This repository of user passwords stored by the Provider is another attractive target for hackers (your password being one of them). Needless to say, Cloud providers need to ensure that the passwords are stored in an encrypted form, and protected by significantly higher security procedures.

The Cloud provider needs to ensure the availability of data to users at all times, and therefore needs to ensure that there is no loss of data even in case of natural events, theft or sabotage. The provider needs to implement procedures for regularly and continuously backing up data to a remote location which is equally well secured as the primary data storage location.

Lastly, Cloud Providers commonly store data from multiple customers on single physical device and within same database. Providers are typically careful to ensure that customer data is segregated in a manner that ensures that the data of one customer is not available accidentally to another. Nevertheless, this is a risk (albeit small) which one assumes when one consigns data to a Cloud Provider.

2.3.3.4.4 Datacenter Personnel

Your data, your passwords, etc. are under the control of the Cloud Provider, which means that at least some personnel within the provider's organization have access to all your data. This is always true, no matter what security policies are implemented by the Cloud Provider. A 'privileged administrator' is a person who has access to the root passwords of the Cloud Provider infrastructure, which in turn means this person potentially has access to data of customers of the Cloud Service Provider.

When your IT infrastructure is housed on your premises and within your control, the 'privileged administrator' is typically someone you personally trust. However, when your data is with a Cloud Service provider, you rely on the provider's policies for recruiting and screening their Privileged Administrator(s). "Ask providers to supply specific information on the hiring and oversight of privileged administrators, and the controls over their access," says a report by Gartner [11].

2.3.3.4.5 Location and Geographical risks

Different countries have different laws and regulations on the ownership of data, its disclosure, privacy requirements, and penalties for offences. If your Cloud provider is based in a country whose laws are different from your own, you assume a risk of your information being subjected to the laws in which your Cloud provider is incorporated.

Your data is at considerably less risk if it is physically located in countries that have strong privacy laws, and strong and functioning legal systems that allow you recourse. Of course with an in house system, this risk does not exist, but even in the case of the Cloud this risk can be eliminated by ensuring that your Cloud Provider stores the data in the same country in which your business is located.

2.3.4 Summary of Security Comparison

To summarize, Cloud providers are likely to be in a better position to protect the data of your practice because they undertake significant investments in technologies, tools and human resources that are required to protect the data. It is hard for a small or mid-sized practice to undertake such a level of investment by itself. Data in transit between your office and the Provider's Datacenter cannot be compromised when it is encrypted and authenticated.

The most significant security risk in using Cloud services is likely to arise from inadvertently compromising the Cloud Service password, by accessing the Cloud Service from locations other than your office, from disgruntled or departed staff members and consultants, from a failure to implement procedures and guidelines for accessing data residing in the cloud or from not exercising due diligence when selecting the cloud vendor.

2.4 ANYTIME, ANYWHERE ACCESS FROM ANY DEVICE

HIPAA & HITECH mandate a degree of information sharing, as well as information access in critical patient scenarios. The value of electronic health records is realized when these records can be made available to attending physicians at the point of care at any geographic location. Thus any healthcare information system needs to ensure the global accessibility of healthcare information in a secure, controlled manner. Secondly, patients need to be given access to their healthcare records via 'Patient Portal'. Thirdly, healthcare information may need to be exchanged with local 'Health Information Exchanges'. All of this means that interoperability, i.e., the ability to exchange and communicate information with other systems and the ability to make information available from anywhere at any time is a key requirement for any system that stores healthcare records.

Cloud service providers devote considerable resources to ensuring that their services are up and running 24x7, i.e., round-the-clock. Occasional 'downtimes' for system upgrades are typically in minutes and are always declared in advance. Cloud-based services can be accessed with a simple browser from any type of computer and from any geographic location. Hence Cloud-based information can be accessed by any individual or their care provider at any time and from any location. (Many Cloud service providers also offer 24x7 'support' to their users either via mail/chat or phone.) If a patient's health records had to be accessed from a random location in a critical scenario, a Cloud-based system is almost certainly guaranteed to deliver that information when and where required.

This round-the-clock availability has a secondary benefit that physicians and nurses no longer need to stay back and work late in the office to finish their work. They can complete some of the IT related work from their homes as well.

Speaking strictly in terms of technology, in-house IT infrastructure can also be accessed from anywhere at any time, using technologies such as Virtual Private Networks (VPN). Virtual Private Networks enable an off-site physician or nurse to remotely and securely log in to the IT infrastructure of the practice, and then complete their work just as they would had they been physically in their office. VPNs require software to be installed on the remote computer (one which is being used by the offsite physician to access the in-house IT). This restricts the type of computers that can be used from remote locations for medical record access. Further, VPNs don't really run well on hand-held devices (when they run at all). So if a physician wants to access in-house electronic health records using a smart phone, there are no guarantees it would be possible with a VPN. Secondly, allowing VPN access to your in-house IT infrastructure entails a security risk. Setting up a secure VPN infrastructure, creating and managing policies for VPNs (assigning/revoking appropriate permissions to various users), creating and enforcing policies for passwords, tracking logs of external access for identifying potential breaches are time consuming tasks that need to be regularly performed when you provide remote access to your in-house IT systems.

Technically, it is also possible to set up a 'Patient portal' on an in-house system. This is done by hosting it on a static IP Address and assigning a domain name to it. Third party care-providers can also access this information in case of emergencies. However, ensuring the security and the 24x7 uptime of the patient portal requires investment of resources and money on part of the healthcare provider. Effectively, this involves putting together an infrastructure equivalent to what Cloud providers have.

Comparison: From a perspective of providing 'Patient portals' and 24x7 location-independent, device-independent access, Cloud-based solutions are better than in-house solutions.

2.5 SYSTEM AUDITS

One significant deterrent to unauthorized access of data in an in-house system is the fact that most organizations install logging/tracking/auditing systems that keep track of all data accesses, information identifying the computer from which each data access request originated, time of access, nature of information accessed, operations performed and other such information. This is easy to do within in-house IT systems that utilize single-sign-on information or identify each computer using its internal IP address.

Some of these details are harder to obtain from Cloud Service Providers. For example, if multiple people within an organization that is behind a NAT (Network Address Translation) firewall access an external Cloud provider, the provider may only see the single 'external' IP address of the organization, and is unable to record the IP address of the specific internal computer where the data request originated. Similarly, if the Cloud service is accessed from dynamically assigned IP address, identifying the originating computer requires cooperation of the Internet Connection Provider. All of this means that tracking usage of a Cloud Service can pose a higher level of logistical difficulty than tracking usage of an in-house system.

Recent regulations require information systems and their usage to be audited periodically. When using a Cloud-based solution, providers should ensure that the necessary audit information will be made available by the Cloud vendor. Figure 2.3 shows the internal and external IPs of a network.

Comparison: An in-house system can be setup to provide more comprehensive auditing and tracking information than a Cloud-based system.

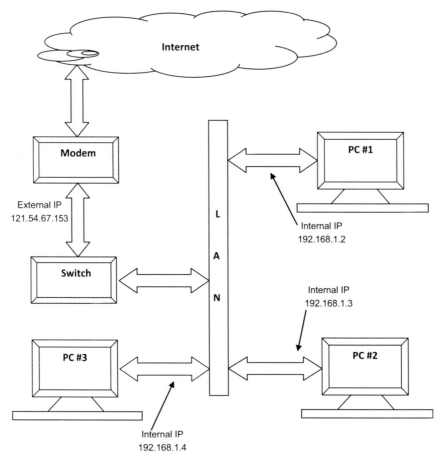

Fig. 2.3 Internal and External IPs.

2.6 BUSINESS MODEL

Any healthcare provider would prefer to work with vendors who can provide solutions and support over a long period of time—many years if not decades. Regulations and requirements change and technologies evolve. Healthcare providers normally expect their vendors to upgrade their solutions to reflect these changes. While selecting an IT system vendor, it is necessary to ensure that the vendor has a stable business model and shall be in a position to support your practice over a long period of time.

Evaluation of the vendor's business stability needs to be done on a case-by-case basis. However, there are certain points that generally apply to in-house systems or Cloud-based systems.

We will cover the Cloud Provider perspective in detail in a subsequent section, but in general, the cost structure of a Cloud-based service provider is likely to be more efficient (less costly) as compared to that of an in-house solution vendor. This is because Cloud-based vendors typically use infrastructure of other Cloud-based vendors to build their services. Secondly, the cost of distribution and support is lesser for Cloud-based providers. On the other hand, the revenue models pursued by Cloud providers involve smaller, periodic income from each customer over a longer period as opposed to larger upfront payments. Due to immense competition to sign up as many subscribers as possible, Cloud Service providers have evolved other innovative business models as well.

Some Cloud Service providers offer their services for free. When a service is free, the Provider typically retains the right to utilize your data in other ways. Some providers display advertisements along with their service and monetize those advertisements. It is not clear at this time if advertisement-driven business models can be sustained over a long period of time in healthcare IT.

Unless a Cloud service provider has a business model that is sustainable and scalable, it poses a risk to your business. If your Cloud Service vendor goes out of business, it can have a potentially catastrophic impact on your practice. Not only does it mean a massive disruption to your business, but you can potentially lose all your data. It is necessary to backup your data independently if you are using a Cloud-based service in order to guard against such a possibility.

If a Cloud Provider is privately owned they are not liable to share financial information with potential subscribers such as you. You must however either ask or estimate the business stability of a prospective provider before consigning all your data to them.

Comparison: Speaking in general terms, packaged software vendors (in-house system providers) have a higher cost associated with running their business, whereas Cloud-based providers see their revenues from a customer realized over a longer period of time. There isn't enough information to determine if Cloud-based healthcare IT systems supported entirely through advertisement revenue are viable.

2.7 CUSTOMIZED SOLUTIONS

Many practices have need for specialized solutions that are either standalone or modifications/enhancements to off-the-shelf products. It is possible to do this when IT is being run in-house—either by seeking software modifications from the solution vendor or by employing third-party consultants to perform the modifications.

On the other hand, a Cloud service provider's business model is based on providing an identical service to many customers. Implicit in this model is the assumption that there are lots of customers looking for the same thing. Cloud service providers typically do not provide an easy way to customize their offering for every customer (although some providers may allow users to customize workflows to certain extent). Few Cloud providers publish an API (i.e., function interfaces) that can be used to build customizations on top of the basic offering. However, there is no guarantee that the customization you seek would be possible, and the process of customization has to rely on the remote support offered by the Cloud provider.

For example, consider a situation where a medical practice needs to generate a very specific type of an analytical report based on information stored in the database. This may not be possible with a Cloud-based service, while it is possible to get a contractor to do it if the database resides within your office.

Comparison: The inability to perform significant customization is a disadvantage of Cloud Services, particularly for those practices that have unusual or unique requirements.

2.8 SYSTEM PERFORMANCE—SPEED, LATENCY, AVAILABILITY

Application latency refers to how fast the software responds to your inputs. Consider a workflow that requires the user to input data sequentially on multiple screens, with inputs being validated by the software as they are entered. The speed with which the software responds to your inputs would have a significant impact on your overall productivity. In-house systems typically have low latency because all data transfer happens over a LAN. This means in-house systems are faster and more responsive. On the other hand, the latency/responsiveness of a Cloud-based service is a function of the speed of your Internet connection at that time. This is because information has to travel back and forth from the remote server over the Internet.

An extreme case is the complete failure of your Internet connection. In this situation, you cannot access your service at all. Running a mission-critical service in the cloud exposes you to the risk that you may potentially be unable to reach the service when you need to. This can be serious when patient care is contingent on the physician's ability to reach the Cloud Service. Near 100% availability is important for critical healthcare applications.

While the quality of internet connections (speeds as well as reliability) have significantly improved, a practice needs to identify and install internet connections of adequate bandwidth (speed) that can deliver acceptable level of performance in terms of system responsiveness and latency. A practice needs to incorporate two types of redundancies—there need to be multiple internet connections from different vendors, and secondly, the bandwidth (speed) of each of the connections should exceed the actual requirement by several times.

Another factor that impacts availability is the planned system 'downtimes'. Both, in-house systems as well as Cloud Services need to be taken down periodically for upgrades, audits or regular maintenance. In case of in-house systems, you can schedule the maintenance timings as per the convenience of your practice. Unfortunately, you have no control on the maintenance schedules of your Cloud service provider.

Most Cloud Service providers schedule their downtimes during intervals of low customer usage (such as nights on weekends) and also provide adequate prior notice of such downtimes. However, there is always the very small likelihood that such a downtime may coincide with the time when you need access to the service.

Comparison: With fast internet connections, the speed of Cloud-based systems can approach those of in-house systems, but in-house systems are theoretically guaranteed to be faster and more responsive. It is best to first evaluate the speed/performance of each Cloud-based system to determine if it is acceptable. Using a Cloud-service opens the possibility (however small) that the service may not be available when you need it—either due to a faulty internet connection or because of a scheduled system downtime.

2.9 VENDOR LOCKIN

Vendor lockin, as the name suggests refers to a situation where it becomes infeasible or extremely hard for a practice to change from a currently used solution from one vendor to another solution from a different vendor. Although a practice is unlikely to change vendors frequently (if ever at all), vendor lockin is not desirable for several reasons. Firstly, it makes it hard for a practice to adopt a different solution—if ever the need arises—such as a new product being introduced with unique features that the practice is looking for. Secondly, it eliminates all competition to the existing vendor and potentially exposes the practice to the risk of excessive pricing or poor support. Thirdly, in the case of the vendor going out of business, it can result in disastrous consequences for your practice.

There is a slightly greater danger of vendor lockin with Cloud-based solutions as opposed to in-house solutions. In the case of in-house solutions, all the data remains under your control at all times, and therefore, migrating this data into another solution is an activity you can undertake with the help of consultants should the need arise. Secondly, it is possible to perform a gradual migration from one provider to another in the case of in-house solutions, again, because all systems involved are under your control.

When it comes to Cloud services, your data resides on the servers that are under the control of the Cloud service provider. Most vendors do not make it simple to transfer all the data from their service to a competing service (for obvious reasons). Therefore it tends to be harder to switch from an existing cloud vendor to a new vendor. Efforts are being made within the Healthcare IT industry to enforce common standards for EMR and other medical data such as CDC & CRC. However there is no guarantee that there would be a way to move data easily between one provider and another. Finally, in case you have developed web-applications based on Cloud services from one vendor, there is no guarantee they would continue to work after you change your cloud vendor.

Comparison: The chances of a vendor lock-in are higher with a Cloud-based provider unless you verify that it is possible to obtain your data from the provider in a standard format at any time.

2.10 SCALABILITY ON DEMAND

If your practice is likely to see a variable level of business around the year, and over the years, your computational requirements won't be constant and are likely to evolve. In such a situation, it is harder to estimate the sort of IT infrastructure one would need in-house. If you underestimate your requirements, it impacts your ability to process patients in a timely fashion. On the other hand, if you overestimate your requirements, your practice ends up paying for material it did not need.

Cloud Services can scale to meet the requirements of your practice virtually on-demand, i.e., without any significant prior work on your part. You can easily add more user accounts if more practitioners join your organization or when more nurses/support staff come on board. Conversely, if you see a reduction in the number of users, you can scale down your utilization of the service. All along, you only pay in proportion to the level of services actually consumed.

Comparison: Easy scalability is a significant benefit of Cloud solutions over in-house solutions for applications in other industry verticals or for healthcare research. Most healthcare providers however, do not see the sort of variation in computing requirements that would make scalability an issue for them.

2.11 COLLABORATION CAPABILITY

As discussed earlier, Cloud Services are accessible anytime, from anywhere via any device. This makes them ideally suited to handle tasks that require collaboration, cooperation or access to common data among multiple entities. When a physician refers a patient to a specialist, both can view the common data stored in the cloud. If health records are maintained in an in-house system with no external access, it is impossible to collaborate on the basis of this information.

Another use-case is the 'eVisit', which enables patients to communicate with their doctors using video conferencing or audio conferencing. Systems that enable such eVisits are usually Cloud-based.

Comparison: Any situation that requires multiple parties to share common resources is best supported by a Cloud-based system.

2.12 CLOUD SERVICE PROVIDER PERSPECTIVE

Just as it is a good idea for a healthcare IT professional to understand the business model of IT vendors, it is also useful to understand the IT vendor perspective when it comes to provisioning of Cloud services. IT vendors find that there are several pros and cons of providing Cloud-based offerings in comparison to in-house offerings. In this section we will review some of these pros and cons.

2.12.1 Cloud Services are easier to market and distribute

Cloud Services are typically marketed over the web—via industry blogs, internet based publications, etc. Some of the most successful Cloud services are marketed 'virally'. Viral marketing is a method of marketing where existing users end up advertising the product to other prospective users during the course of using the product.

Many Cloud Service Providers allow prospective users to try the service for a limited time with no fees, thereby eliminating the need for sales staff doing on-site demonstrations.

The Cloud Service distribution model is direct-to-consumer model. There are no distributors or agents involved, and a practice can sign up directly with the Provider whenever the practice is ready. There is no 'installation' involved either. In other words, marketing and distributing a Cloud service is substantially cheaper and easier than marketing and distributing software meant for in-house installation.

This levels the playing field for companies with great products but without the marketing reach to compete effectively. The Cloud model therefore makes it possible for great products from smaller companies to reach you directly. This would not have been possible earlier with packaged software.

2.12.2 Cloud services are easier to support

Customer support can be a significant cost for vendors providing in-house software—although vendors do often bill customers for the support costs. Providing customer support is people-intensive and requires continuous training of resources. To trouble-shoot in-house software, support staff needs access to the internal IT of the customer. When remote access is not possible, travel becomes essential, thereby increasing the time taken to fix the problem. When support is charged to the customer, it is an expense the customer typically resents.

Supporting a Cloud-based offering on the other hand is much simpler. The support personnel can instantly see what is wrong by reviewing the server logs/databases and either fix the problem or provide the necessary support on the spot. This is convenient not only for the provider but also for the customer.

2.12.3 Version release and maintaining backward compatibility is easier in the Cloud

Software vendors release periodic upgrades of their products (either when problems are fixed or new features or functionality is added). When this happens, existing installations of the software need to be upgraded. Each time there is a version upgrade, backward compatibility needs to be maintained to ensure that previous work of users is not lost. Secondly it is in the interest of the Software vendor to ensure that all users migrate to later versions as soon as possible, but ensuring this is not easy. The overall process of version upgradation in the case of installed software is cumbersome and time consuming, and it also needs the cooperation of the customer. Software upgrades for packaged software are therefore released usually about twice every year.

However, in the case of Cloud Services releasing a new version is easy and inexpensive for the Provider. Only the software on the servers needs to be upgraded, and every single customer automatically begins using the new version when they log in next. Maintaining backward compatibility for all users is also easy. This makes it possible for Cloud Providers to introduce software upgrades much more frequently, often once a week. This means Cloud Providers are likely to fix issues much faster when they are reported.

2.12.4 Cloud Services are easier to offer

Software as a Service (Cloud Service) is easier to deploy, distribute, and support. For this reason, many software vendors will gradually move to delivering their solutions as Cloud Services. Secondly, Cloud technologies have made it possible for smaller companies to compete on an equal footing with larger, more established players. Cloud Services are hence the preferred mechanism for smaller companies and startups to bring their solutions to the market.

Comparison: From a vendor perspective, it is much easier to launch, support and upgrade Cloud-based solutions than packaged software. Cloud-based solutions are also easier to market and distribute.

2.13 PERCEPTIONS

In the previous sections of this chapter, we have covered the advantages and disadvantages of Cloud-based solutions when compared to in-house solutions.

Several organizations have conducted surveys of CIOs and other key decision-makers, and the findings of those surveys mirror the points we have already covered.

In the IDC survey conducted in 2009 [1] for example, the top three benefits of Cloud solutions as perceived by respondents were:

1) Usage-linked payment ('pay-as-you-go')
2) Ease of deployment
3) Monthly payment

The top three drawbacks of Cloud solutions as per the same survey were:

1) Security
2) Availability
3) Performance

Note that the above survey was not specifically focused on the healthcare industry, but covered a general sample of users.

As per the Mimecast survey referred earlier [3], the top two reasons why users adopted Cloud-based solutions were:

1) Cost
2) Agility

The top two concerns that represent a barrier to cloud adoption are:

1) Security concerns
2) Loss of control

[5] is an excellent reference that contains an overview of the perceived barriers to EMR adoption. Cloud-based systems could help overcome some of the perceptions listed therein.

2.14 SUMMARY

It is clear that Cloud-based solutions can be easily and cost-effectively adopted by small physician practices. These practices however need to ensure that the specific solution they adopt provides safeguards that address the vulnerabilities of Cloud-based solutions. These practices also need to put in place policies that govern the access and usage of Cloud services by their staff. Finally, redundancy in internet infrastructure is a must in order to minimize the chances of solution non-availability.

REFERENCES

[1] http://blogs.idc.com/ie/?p=730
[2] http://www.gartner.com/it/page.jsp?id=1035013
[3] http://www.mimecast.com/cloudsurvey/
[4] http://www.aafp.org/online/en/home/publications/news/news-now/practice-management/20080626ehr-survey.html
[5] EHR Adoption: A Barrier Analysis, Fabio Sabogal, 2004, DOQ-IT.
[6] Applied Cryptography, Bruce Schneier, John Wiley & Sons, 1996
[7] Security Engineering: A Guide to Building Dependable Distrubuted Systems, Ross Anderson, John Wiley & Sons, 2001.
[8] http://csrc.nist.gov/publications/secpubs/web-secvul.pdf
[9] http://www.coresecurity.com/content/Operation-Aurora-Attacks
[10] http://docs.sun.com/source/816-6156-10/contents.htm
[11] http://www.gartner.com/DisplayDocument?id=685308

CHAPTER 3

Cloud Technologies

We mentioned in an earlier chapter that Cloud-based services are more than just outsourced application hosting. There is substantial technology innovation that makes the delivery of Cloud services feasible at relatively low price points. Some of the key technology innovations have to do with optimizing the utilization of computing resources, optimizing data storage and retrieval, information backup and replication, ensuring security of information and so on.

A user of Cloud-based services, per se, need not be concerned with the underlying technologies that make Cloud Services possible. However, understanding these technologies gives the user a much better idea of how his data is processed and stored in the cloud.

Three fundamental aspects pertaining to Cloud-based services are noteworthy:

1) Browser-based applications, i.e., applications that run entirely within a browser

2) Optimal use of server resources, i.e., partitioning, scaling, virtualization and multi-tenancy.

3) Datacenters, modern standards and their management.

In this chapter we will cover these key aspects.

3.1 BROWSER-BASED APPLICATIONS

Browser-based applications, i.e., applications that run entirely within browsers are different from traditional applications which either run natively on computers (most users are familiar with these) or are structured as 'client-server' applications. In this section, we will first review these traditional applications which will provide us the background to understand how browser applications are different.

3.1.1 Native Applications

Native Applications are those that run entirely on the computer on which they are invoked (launched). A native application uses only the computing resources and storage of the computer which was used to launch the application. For example, if you have a copy of Microsoft Office installed on your PC and launch Microsoft Word, it uses the CPU and memory of your computer to perform all the operations required to properly run Microsoft Word. The files you save are also saved on the hard-disk of the same PC. Microsoft Word is therefore a 'Native application', i.e., it 'runs natively' on your computer.

Native applications have several drawbacks. Firstly, they are not suitable for situations where collaboration between multiple individuals is essential. Consider for example a practice that has several doctors, nurses and other staff members involved in the delivery of care to patients. It is likely that different individuals may update different portions of the patient records—for example staff members may update information obtained from lab tests, doctors may update prescriptions, and so on. However, the practice would want to consolidate and maintain together all the information about a patient—no matter who enters it. This way, any doctor or nurse can see exactly the same consolidated records of any patient at a particular time. This consolidation is best done by storing all of the patients' information in a single storage repository by the practice. Anyone who updates the information directly updates it in the repository and anyone who wants to look up the information looks it up from that same repository.

Having pieces of patient information reside and be managed on different computers by native applications would not work because updates made on one computer would not effectively propagate to other computers. Consequently, there would be no guarantee that everyone was seeing identical patient information. Native applications are therefore not suitable for situations where multiple entities have to touch (modify or view) common data.

The second drawback of native applications is that they are inefficient from a point of view of hardware utilization. Each computer running a native application has to be a machine powerful enough to handle entirely by itself the most computationally intensive task within the application. For example consider an application that requires computationally intensive analysis to be run on data occasionally. If this analysis were performed by a native application, each of the individual computers would need to be powerful enough to support the required level of computational workload. This means the practice would need to invest in multiple, powerful machines only in order to support computationally intensive analysis which is infrequently done. It would be a lot more efficient if each of the users were to access a single, powerful, central computer to run the analysis when required.

Thirdly, upgrade and maintenance of native applications is more time consuming because the upgrades have to be performed on several individual computers.

These drawbacks of native applications are overcome by Client Server Systems.

3.1.2 Client Server Systems

As the name suggests, Client Server systems involve a powerful central computer ('powerful' refers to its ability to perform relatively higher number of computations, 'central' refers to its direct accessibility by multiple other computers), called the Server. In addition, they involve multiple other computers (called 'Clients') within the practice, which are used by individuals to connect to this Server over a Local Area Network (LAN). The Server often has a Database installed on it or connected to it.

Most software modules run on the Server (Server software) while some of the modules run on the Client computers (Client Software). The purpose of the Client Software is:

1) To establish a connection with the Server software for to and fro data transfer from the Server.
2) To enable the individual to enter data and commands. The entered data and commands are communicated to the Server. The Server processes the data and the commands, and it usually

involves initiating a computation or storage or retrieval of data from the database connected to the server.

3) To display the results returned by the Server.

It is possible that some minor operations are performed on the client computers as well, although the bulk of storage and computation is performed on the Server.

Because all data is stored in a central database, any individual from any computer accesses exactly the same up-to-date data at any time. Secondly, the Server is typically a powerful machine capable of performing complex computations fast. The Server supports simultaneous connections from multiple clients, and can execute requests from multiple such clients simultaneously. At such times, the Server resources (CPU power, memory) are divided among these multiple tasks. If too many clients simultaneously initiate tasks on the server, the server appears to slow down for each of the clients because of the division of resources mentioned above. While planning the infrastructure, typical simultaneous loads on the server are estimated, and servers that can deliver an acceptable level of performance for this estimated load are installed. You can also set up the system so that the number of simultaneous connections to the server is limited.

The data in the central database is backed-up periodically on a device such as a tape drive or any other backup storage. Figure 3.1 shows the client server network over the LAN.

Upgrading the software requires an upgrade to the Server software, and also an upgrade to the client software running on each of the individual computers.

Client and Server systems are developed for particular platforms. It is possible though that the Client Software and the Server Software are developed for two different platforms. For example, the client software may be developed for Microsoft Windows XP platform whereas the Server software runs on Redhat Linux. Client Server software need not run on a LAN. It can run on a WAN (Wide area network) as well. Most enterprise software traditionally is designed as Client Server software, and is the primary alternative to Cloud-based Services that are the subject of this book.

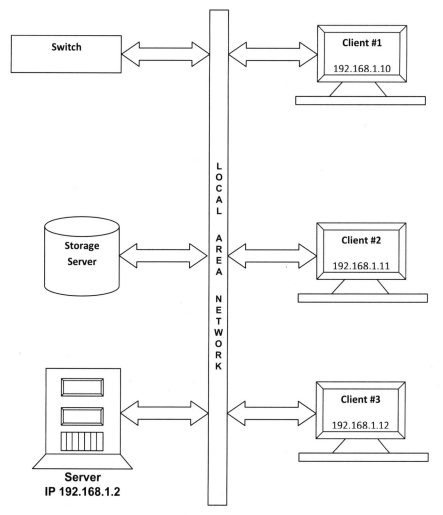

Fig. 3.1 Client Server Topology.

3.1.3 Browser based applications

Browser based applications are applications that run from within Internet Browsers, i.e., they are launched from within a browser by accessing a web server at a particular internet address. The information sent by the Web Server is displayed by the Browser. Users can enter data and provide commands via the Browser which communicates the entered data and commands to the Web Server. In response, the Web Server sends back new information to be displayed to the Browser.

Browser applications are conceptually similar to Client Server applications, but there are two specific characteristics:

1) As the name suggests, Browser based applications can *only* be invoked from inside a standard browser. The Browser performs the functions performed by the 'client' in a traditional client-server application. This includes the communication with the server which is done using a standard protocol called the HTTP (Hypertext Transfer Protocol) or a secure version of it called the HTTPS (Hypertext Transfer Protocol—Secure). Secondly, the browser performs the function of rendering user-interfaces that are compliant with a standard language called HTML (Hypertext Markup Language).

2) The Client and the Server are not (necessarily) a part of a Local Area Network. They can be geographically distant, and communication between them happens over the Internet. Servers are accessed with a globally applicable Internet Address or a mapped URL.

Browser-based applications make it possible for Software to be delivered as a 'Service'. Most of the computations are performed on the Web Server, and the same Web Server can support several simultaneous connections from customers. Virtually all computers/operating systems include a browser, which means the Service can be accessed from anywhere and from any device.

We examine the role of the Browser and the Web Server in slightly greater detail.

3.1.3.1 Internet Browser

Internet Browsers are Native applications that are capable of:

1) Communicating with Internet Servers to send and receive information including
   a. Sending HTTP requests for information to any web-accessible internet address
   b. Rendering (i.e., displaying) the information received in HTML format
2) Providing users the ability to navigate from one internet location to another.
3) Running (executing) code within them to perform certain basic operations.

Well known examples of browsers are Microsoft's Internet Explorer and Mozilla's Firefox.

Wikipedia [1] defines Browsers as "a software application for retrieving, presenting, and traversing information resources on the World Wide Web. An 'information resource' is identified by a Uniform Resource Identifier (URI) and may be a web page, image, video, or other piece of content. Hyperlinks present in resources enable users to easily navigate their browsers to related resources."

3.1.3.2 The Web Server

In the case of Browser based applications, the server is a 'Web server'. The primary functions of the Web server are

1) To receive and interpret HTTP requests over the Internet from clients (usually Internet Browsers)
2) To fulfill those requests by sending back to the originating client data in the HTML format.

In the simplest scenario, the request is fulfilled by sending a HTML file resident on the Web Server back to the browser as a response. However, it is also possible to write small programs or 'scripts' that govern the behavior of the Web server (i.e., define how the web-server processes specific requests received from the browsers). Cloud Service Providers can write 'scripts' that perform certain actions in response to requests received from the browsers. These programs can also access databases that are resident on computers connected to the server. PHP is an example of a language that is used for writing Web Server Scripts.

Examples of Web Servers are Microsoft's IIS, Apache from Apache Foundation, etc.

3.1.3.3 The Communication Process

Cloud Services (like any website) are accessible with their URL (Unique Resource Locator) on the Internet. When the user types the URL of a Cloud Service in the browser, the browser first queries a Domain Name Server (DNS) to look up the Internet Protocol Address (IP Address) of the server that the URL points to. The IP Address uniquely points to the physical server on which the Cloud Service is located. The browser then sends the request for data to the server at that IP address. This request is made in the Hypertext Transfer Protocol (HTTP) format. In response, the Server sends back information to the browser in the HTML (Hypertext Markup Language) format, which the browser interprets and displays as a web-page. As the user continues to navigate (i.e., perform actions within the web-pages successively rendered by the browser), the browser keeps sending appropriate HTTP requests to the server and the server keeps responding to those requests with HTML data. Each such response from the Server results in the browser displaying updated information to the user.

Web-pages rendered by the browser need not necessarily be plain text. They can contain elements for user interaction such as text boxes where users can type in text, drop down menus, buttons for user selection, and so on. Any actions performed by the user using these elements are also communicated to the Server by the browser as a part of the HTTP request.

A secure version of the HTTP protocol is the Secure HTTP, also called the HTTPS protocol. The purpose of the secure protocol is to ensure the authentication of the client and the server, and the confidentiality of data transmitted in either direction. In this protocol, the following happens:

1) When the browser sends its first request to the server, the server authenticates itself to the browser by means of a 'certificate'. This certificate assures the browser that the server is indeed the right server, i.e., the server that the browser intended to reach. Such upfront server validation is important. For example, if the user was entering medical data into a browser, he would need the guarantee that the data would reach the intended server (i.e., the server of the particular Cloud-service provider) and not any other malicious server.

2) The server and the browser exchange a cryptographic key which is used to encrypt all subsequent communication between the browser and the server. Again, encryption is important because the Internet is a public medium and sensitive data such as medical data should always be securely communicated in an encrypted fashion over the Internet.

3) HTTPS communication also includes a cryptographic hash as a part of all data communicated each way. The receiver (server

or browser) recomputes the hash of the received data and compares it with the hash received from the sender (browser or server respectively). This comparison ensures the integrity of the communicated data, i.e., it ensures that the data hasn't being modified in transit over the internet.

Once the initial handshake is completed, all subsequent data transfer (both ways) in that session is hashed and encrypted, ensuring its confidentiality and integrity. The URLs of Cloud-based healthcare services that are accessed over HTTPS protocol are typically prefixed with an https://. The details of the HTTPS protocol are provided in an appendix.

Internet Browser security settings often need to be adjusted so as to allow web applications to run within them. Browsers cannot perform certain operations such as accessing local resources or data on your computer unless explicitly permitted by you via the settings. Running web applications that require access to local resources typically requires you to relax the privacy and security settings in your browser.

Browser plugins are scripts that execute within the browser. Some web applications require you to download and install such plugins into your browser so as to facilitate functioning of the web application. These plugins are updated/upgraded as required by the web application directly. One of the best known examples of a plugin is the Adobe Flash plugin, which enables users to run several applications that are written in the Flex language.

3.1.3.4 Example of a simple web application

Consider a web program that allows the user to look up her Electronic Health Records by entering her Social Security Number and name. When the user types the URL of the Web Program in her browser, she sees a page where she can type her Name and Social Security Number and press the Enter button. On pressing the Enter Button, the Browser securely communicates this information (Name and Social Security Number) to the Web Server. Upon receiving the HTTPS request containing the name and Social Security Number, the Web program looks up its database for the Health Record corresponding to that Social Security Number, then verifies that the name in the Health record matches the name supplied by the user. If it matches, the Records are sent back to the Browser securely in the form of a web-page. The Browser displays the webpage containing the Health Record to the user.

When complex Web applications have to be developed, programmers often use an 'Application Server' in addition to a Web Server. The Application Server communicates with the Web Server and either runs on the same physical computer or another computer within the service-provider infrastructure. The Application Server provides the application developer with a framework for writing complex web-applications. These web-applications running on the Application Server can be used to define the behavior of the Web Server in response to HTTP requests received by the Web Server. Figure 3.2 shows the interaction between the Application server and the Web server.

The primary advantages of using an Application Server are

   a. It provides a framework for writing complex applications. It helps the developer centralize all the business logic, which also makes it easier to upgrade the applications.

   b. It typically helps improve performance of the application.

Examples of Application Servers are: Apache Tomcat, Websphere from IBM, Weblogic from Oracle, JBoss from Red Hat, etc.

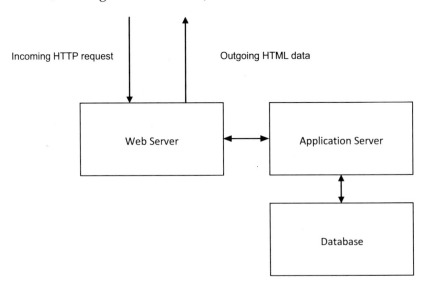

Fig. 3.2 Block Diagram of Web Server/Application Server.

3.1.3.5 *Common Web-application Technologies*

The following are some of the commonly used web application development technologies [2] [3]:

1) *Javascript* is a scripting language that works with HTML to enhance web pages and make them more interactive. These scripts are executed on the client side

2) *PHP* is a popular language to create web sites. PHP is an interpreted language and is executed on server side.

3) *PERL* is a server side scripting language. Perl scripts are text files which are executed by an "interpreter" on the server.

4) JavaServer Pages (JSP) is a Java technology that helps software developers serve dynamically generated web pages based on HTML, XML, or other document types.

5) ASP.NET is a web application framework developed and marketed by Microsoft to allow programmers to build dynamic web sites, web applications and web services.

3.2 SERVER RESOURCE OPTIMIZATION

Cloud Service Providers see variable level of utilization of their services. This variability has two components. Firstly, the number of simultaneous users accessing the service is different at different times. For example, for typical business applications, the number of simultaneous users is likely to be much higher during work hours than it is on weekend nights. Secondly, the processing and storage resources required by any particular user are never constant. A Cloud Service infrastructure needs to be designed to deal with a variable level of computational load. In other words, Cloud Services need to be 'scalable'. Ensuring this scalability requires the deployment of specific technologies.

As mentioned earlier, many simultaneous users are likely to be accessing the service at any given time. The Cloud Service infrastructure needs to ensure separation between the data (and processes) of different users who are simultaneously accessing the service. Data of one subscriber should obviously not be visible to another. Similarly, any issues with a process being run by one user should not interfere with the smooth operation of the process being run by another user. For example, a computationally intensive process initiated by one user should not slow down the operations of other users.

From a point of view of economics, it is impossible for the Cloud provider to provide separate physical machines and storage for each user. Therefore, the Cloud Provider needs to deploy technology that allows the simultaneous running of multiple independent processes on the same physical hardware in a way that they do not interfere with each other. Also, the Cloud provider needs to implement technologies that ensure that data of one subscriber is not visible to another subscriber even though both of their data is stored on the same physical storage. Apportioning physical resources among multiple simultaneous users in a way that they do not interfere with one another is called resource partitioning.

Technologies for scaling and resource partitioning are at the heart of Cloud Services because without these technologies, the Cloud business model would not be feasible. In order to meet their specific goals, Cloud Providers can choose from a number of available technologies as appropriate.

3.2.1 Load Balancing

In the context of hosted applications, Load Balancing denotes a mechanism for rational or even distribution of load across multiple physical resources, such as servers, storage devices or communication links. The hosting infrastructure typically involves multiple instances of similar devices such as multiple servers, multiple data links, multiple storage devices and so on. This is not only for the sake of redundancy or failsafe operation, but also because a single physical device may not be adequate to support the expected load. Implementing Load Balancing ensures optimal utilization of all resources, maximizes speed of execution and enhances reliability of the overall system. The Load Balancer is either a software or hardware that matches every need for a resource with an appropriate physical instance of that resource.

A server load balancer is responsible for balancing the load of incoming requests among a bank of physical servers. Any incoming HTTP request first hits the server load balancer, which then decides the precise physical server to forward the request to for fulfillment. The criteria employed by the load balancer to select the precise server may vary. For example, the load balancer may simply direct each request to a random server, or may assign requests to the servers in a round-robin fashion. For applications that require a preservation of state (context) among successive requests from the same browser, it makes sense for the load balancer to direct each request from a particular user session to the same physical server. The load balancer can do this on the basis of the IP address of the machine from where the requests originated. When a server processes a request, it sends the response back to the Load balancer which then forwards it to the originating client (browser). By effectively distributing the workload associated with processing incoming HTTP requests among various physical servers, the load balancer ensures even utilization of resources. Furthermore, performance is maximized because no single server sees an inordinate computational load. If one server fails, the load balancer automatically stops forwarding requests to the failed server, thereby ensuring a level of fault tolerance in the system. Physical servers can be added or removed from behind the load balancer, thereby providing the ability to scale the infrastructure in tune with the demand. Figure 3.3 shows the server load balancer configuration.

In a similar way, a storage load balancer is necessary when multiple physical storage devices are to be used for storing data. A storage load balancer sits in front of the physical storage devices and directs the data to be stored to one of the multiple storage devices. Such a distribution optimizes the average read and write times associated with storage operations.

Load balancers make it possible for a Provider to add or remove additional servers or storage devices and therefore ensure that infrastructure scales up and down with the demand. Further details can be found in [4], [5].

3.2.2 Virtualization

Virtualization is the process of abstracting the logical resources as seen by the user from the actual physical resources. In other words, virtualization allows a single physical resource to be used like multiple resources or multiple physical resources to be used like a single resource.

There are several types of virtualization, depending on the nature of the physical resource that is 'virtualized'.

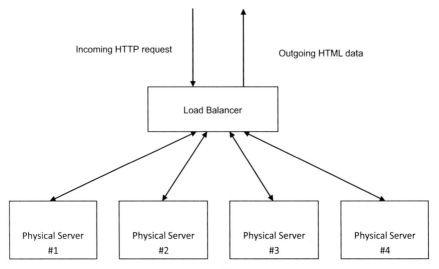

Fig. 3.3 Block Diagram of Server Load Balancing.

3.2.2.1 Server Virtualization

In this type of virtualization, a single physical server is converted into multiple logical servers. In other words, virtualization creates silos on a single physical server, such that within each silo, a different operating system or process can run independently of what operating systems or processes are running in other silos.

It is common for most organizations to use different physical servers for various functions such as Mail, Collaboration, CRM and so on. Each of these servers is typically utilized to only between 5–20% of its capacity, according to industry estimates. Virtualization allows all of these servers to run on a single machine, and thereby not only save significantly on infrastructure costs, but also allow more efficient utilization of resources.

Server virtualization also allows the opposite to happen—it also allows multiple physical servers to be viewed as a single server for running an Operating system or an application. Some processes (analytics for example) are so computationally intensive that running them on a single server would take an inordinate amount of time. In such a situation it is useful to divide the computational load among multiple servers so as to complete the task in shorter time. By employing virtualization, the analytical program can run in a way whereby the computations are performed in parallel on different physical servers. It is important to note that no modifications are required to the analytical program. The task of assigning computations to different physical servers and recombining answers is handled by the Virtualization Engine. To the user, it is as if the program had run on a single physical server— only faster.

Server virtualization therefore provides the ability to make either fractional or multiple computational resources available to any program, without any modifications to the program.

3.3.2.2 Storage Virtualization

In this type of virtualization, a single storage device is converted into multiple logical storage devices, or vice-versa, i.e., multiple storage devices are converted into a single logical storage device. A simple example of storage virtualization is the partitioning of a single hard-disk into multiple disks so that each of them can be treated independently—they can be formatted independently for example.

When large amount of data has to be stored, it is impossible to store it on a single device whose capacity is smaller than the amount of data that has to be stored. It is necessary to be able to add physical storage devices as needed over a period of time, without having to make changes to the software or the process configuration. With virtualization, it is possible to seamlessly add or remove physical storage devices as required by the process. The program or the user of the program does not know on which particular storage device a particular record of data exists, nor is it material to him.

In the Cloud services scenario, the users may potentially need to store vast quantities of data. Data of multiple users may be stored in a single database, and hence the size of the database grows over time. Storage virtualization makes it possible for the service provider to easily add storage devices to keep up with the increasing requirement.

3.3.2.3 Network Virtualization

Network virtualization allows the user to split a single communication link into separate channels assigned to different processes. Conversely, it also allows the user to consolidate multiple communication links into a single logical link of higher bandwidth. Both of these are important in a Cloud service scenario.

Multiple processes from multiple users access the Cloud Service over a common communication pipe (the connection from the Cloud Server to the Service Provider's ISP). The Provider would want to avoid a situation where a single user's process consumes most of the bandwidth to the detriment of other user processes. It is not acceptable to have a single user 'hog' the bandwidth in a manner that slows down the connection for other users. With virtualization it is possible for the Provider to 'split' his total bandwidth into multiple logical links of lower bandwidth each so that each individual process is assigned only a single logical link. This restricts the bandwidth usage of that user to only a slice of the overall bandwidth.

Conversely, there is a also a need to combine several physical links into a single logical link. Any Cloud Service Provider typically has multiple communication pipes to the Internet for the reason of a failsafe operation. In normal times, the Provider would like to utilize the sum total of the bandwidth provided by the pipes. Of course the Provider would not like to go through the exercise of apportioning different users to different pipes because failure of a single pipe would require the Provider to distribute the users on that pipe to other functional pipes. Network virtualization makes it easy for the Provider, because it allows the Provider to treat all the available pipes as a single communication pipe of consolidated capacity. When a single pipe fails, users are automatically accommodated on the remaining functional pipes.

3.2.3 How Server Virtualization works

Virtualization is made possible by software called the 'Hypervisor' that resides between the hardware and the operating systems thereby isolating the two from each other. On one hand, the Hypervisor can logically consolidate multiple computers into a single large processor of consolidated capacity and consolidated disk space. On the other hand, it can divide this consolidated processing capacity into pieces that it can assign to each operating system. Thus it is the Hypervisor that performs the allocation of available hardware resources to the operating system, or multiple operating systems as the case may be. The hypervisor also keeps each operating system independent of the others. Thirdly, the hypervisor continually monitors the available physical resources. As various processes run within each Operating system, the Hypervisor assigns available resources to the process that requires them. Figure 3.4 shows a block diagram of the hypervisor.

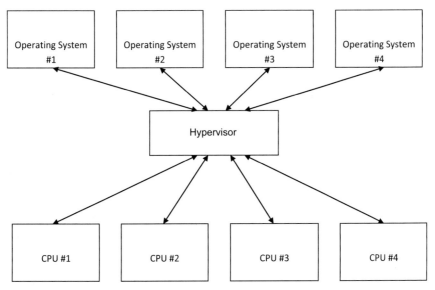

Fig. 3.4 Block Diagram of Hypervisor.

3.2.4 Benefits of Virtualization

Virtualization brings significant operating benefits to the Cloud Service Provider thereby substantially reducing the cost of providing the services. Virtualization is primarily responsible for enabling the Cloud Service business model that allows providers to provide on-demand, pay-as-you-go services for small monthly fees.

Virtualization allows Providers to divert physical resources as required to those subscriber processes that actually need them at a given point in time.

1) Virtualization enables providers to run processes of multiple subscribers on a single physical machine, thereby saving not only on additional servers, networking and storage equipment, but also on the associated overheads and administrative costs.

2) Virtualization enables the Provider to isolate various subscriber processes from each other so that they run independently of each other.

3) Virtualization creates an infrastructure that is fault tolerant, adaptable and therefore easier to manage for the Provider.

4) Virtualization allows the Cloud Provider to scale his business easily in conjunction with the subscriber demand.

References [6], [7] may be consulted for more information on virtualization.

3.2.5 Multi-tenancy

Just as Virtualization can partition a physical server into multiple logical servers, Multi-tenancy is the principal of architecting applications such that a single instance of the application running on the server is visible as separate instances of the same application for each of the clients connected to it. Multi-tenancy requires partitioning the configuration settings and data of each client so as to support them independently with the same application instance.

Multi-tenancy is different from virtualization (where the physical machine is partitioned to appear as separate physical machines). In the case of multi-tenancy, although different clients are accessing the same application on the same operating system, and have their data stored within the same database, they are cannot see each other's data and can have their own application configurations.

Multi-tenancy also offers some of the same advantages that Virtualization does. For example, by allowing multiple clients to access the same application on the server, it reduces hardware and maintenance costs and simplifies the process of releasing new versions of the application.

3.3 THE DATACENTER

Cloud Service Provider's infrastructure is usually housed in a Datacenter, and the Datacenter is where the user's data is processed and stored. To understand how secure your Cloud data is, one needs to understand the working of a Datacenter.

Modern Datacenters are extraordinarily designed—with the purpose of protecting your data and keeping it accessible at all times. Without the high availability and high reliability afforded by modern Datacenters, providing Cloud services would not be a viable business simply because customers would not subscribe to an unreliable service. Designing and Operating Datacenters is a field in itself, and there are numerous standards and guidelines impacting virtually every aspect of a Datacenter, including its design, construction, and operation. For example, the Telecommunications Industry Association (TIA) has defined guidelines for Datacenters in [8]. TIA defines guidelines for four different levels of Datacenters— Tier 1 being the lowest, and applicable to a basic server room, and Tier 4 being the highest—for those Datacenters that house highly mission critical data. Another set of guidelines, particularly for a Datacenter's physical security are found in [9].

Most modern Datacenters conform to standard guidelines such as those referenced above. Some of the design considerations for Datacenters are as below:

1) Datacenters are typically located in places where the risk of natural disasters (such as earthquakes, floods, hurricanes, etc) and man-made disasters (such as riots, explosions, etc.) is minimal. They are located in places with abundant availability of resources such as water and electricity.

2) Buildings used to house Datacenters typically do not house other offices and businesses. The area around the Datacenter is usually well lit and easy to monitor. It is easy to control access into the premises where the Datacenter is housed.

3) Datacenters have areas with raised flooring where servers are housed in racks. There are separate ducts through which power cables and networking cables to the servers are laid out.

4) Datacenters have air-conditioning that maintains the temperature and humidity within limits that suit the optimal working of the servers.

5) Datacenters have multiple levels of physical security, including armed guards, video surveillance, biometric access controls, etc. that make unauthorized access virtually impossible.

6) Datacenters have assured continuous electric supply. They have power backups with instant failover, comprising uninterrupted power supplies and diesel generators.

7) Datacenters have state of art fire prevention and fire protection systems. This involves fire detectors, sprinkler systems, fire retarding systems including clean agent gaseous systems.

From a networking perspective:

1) Datacenters have high-bandwidth data pipes with multiple levels of redundancy. This ensures high speed connectivity even if one of the links goes down.
2) Internally, Datacenters have all the elements installed that are required to continually run Intranet services. These are high quality, high throughput systems.
3) Datacenters implement the most advanced Network security tools including intrusion detection, firewalls, antivirus systems, and systems that guard against spamming, Denial of Service Attacks, and all known malware.

Lastly,

1) Datacenters employ qualified system administrators normally after a thorough check of their background.
2) Datacenters have systems and processes in place to support smooth functioning 24x7 and throughout the year.
3) Datacenters have disaster recovery plans, in case accidents happen in spite of all the precautions taken.

It is a fact that the data in a modern Datacenter is most likely to be better protected than it is in a typical medical practice. It is not viable for a typical medical practice to operate at the level of security, reliability and availability at which a modern Datacenter operates.

3.4 PRIVATE CLOUDS

'Private Cloud' is terminology used to describe a Cloud Service type of an infrastructure put in place for the use of a single organization. The 'Datacenter' for the private cloud could be located physically within the organization itself, or in rented space at a regular Datacenter. For large organizations such as large hospitals, that have the scale and level of usage to justify such an expense, it is sometimes attractive to deploy software in a manner similar to a Cloud Service, but without the risk of dealing with an entity that is not a part of the organization. The software is built with technologies similar to those used for regular Cloud-based offerings. But the infrastructure (servers, networking, storage devices, etc.) is owned by and under control of the organization. The organization also makes the policies for personnel and procedures for use of the private Cloud services. Such an in-house deployment of information technology which leverages Cloud Technologies is referred to as a Private Cloud. Sometimes, the Private Cloud is deployed only on the internal network, and is not accessible over the Internet. The accessibility depends on the nature of the applications provided from the Private Cloud.

The Private Cloud entails incurring the cost disadvantages associated with in-house IT, since you have to put up the entire infrastructure for the use of your organization alone. On the other hand the benefit of the Private Cloud is the security it offers. The Private Cloud is subject to the policies of the organization, just as its operation is under the organization's control. Therefore, data really never 'leaves' your premises. This addresses the key concern pertaining to (public) Cloud services, namely, control over the data.

The Private Cloud option however, is really an option only for larger organizations who can afford to undertake the expense involved.

An infrastructure that has elements in the Public Cloud and the Private Cloud is referred to as a Hybrid Cloud.

3.5 SAAS MODEL

The traditional SaaS (Software as a Service) model is used by several vendors of healthcare IT solutions to provide services to their customers. In this model:

1) The solution is installed and hosted on servers which are housed at a Datacenter, rather than on-premise.

2) The solution can be accessed by the practice remotely over the internet, using technologies such as Virtual Private Networks (VPN) or similar remote-access technologies (rather than a browser). All data processing and storage happens on the servers in the Datacenter.

3) The billing model is 'pay-as-you go'. There is little or no upfront fee, and users are charged monthly for using the solution.

VPN (virtual private network) is an example of remote access technology. A VPN (virtual private network) is a computer network that is layered on top of other underlying computer networks. It allows for transfer of data between two private networks in such a way that the data travelling over the VPN is not visible to or accessible to the underlying computer networks. VPNs are typically used to create a secure connection between two geographically distant LANs (Local Area Networks) over the internet. When a computer connects to a LAN over a VPN, it is effectively treated a part of the same LAN. Figure 3.5 shows the establishment of VPN over the cloud.

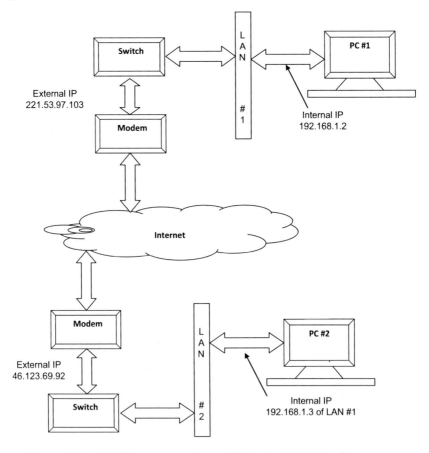

Fig. 3.5 When PC #2 is connected over VPN to LAN #1, it is obtains an Internal IP of LAN #1.

There are some technological differences between such a solution, and the Cloud solutions discussed in earlier sections. However, from a user perspective, the only difference is really the usage of a VPN rather than a browser to access the servers.

For this reason, such SaaS solutions are also often considered as 'Cloud solutions'. This is particularly true in the healthcare industry where a number of vendors offer hosted solutions for monthly fees.

REFERENCES

[1] http://en.wikipedia.org/wiki/Web_browser

[2] http://www.binarysec.com/cms/docs/resources/glossary/p-s.html

[3] http://www.greenwebdesign.com/Glossary-Of-Technical-Terms.htm

[4] *Server Load balancing*, Tony Bourke, O'Reilly Media, 2001.

[5] http://www.loadbalancing.org/

[6] *Virtualization, A Beginner's guide*, Nelson Ruest, Danielle Ruest, McGraw Hill Osborne Media.

[7] *Storage Virtualization: Technologies for Simplifying Data Storage and Management*, Tom Clark, Addison-Wesley, 2005.

[8] http://www.adc.com/us/en/Library/Literature/102264AE.pdf

[9] http://grouper.ieee.org/groups/802/3/10GBT/public/nov03/diminico_1_1103.pdf

SECTION II

CLOUD SERVICES FOR HEALTHCARE IT

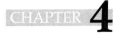

CHAPTER 4

Cloud-based Solutions for Healthcare IT

Cloud-based systems are being used in a number of industry verticals for applications such as Enterprise backup and storage, Productivity tools (Word Processing, spreadsheets, presentation, collaboration), Accounting and Financial applications, ERP, and so on with success. Businesses, in particular smaller businesses have been using such Cloud-based solutions for several years now. The fact that Cloud-based services cost significantly less and require virtually no upfront expense makes Cloud services particularly attractive to this user group. Reported cases of security breaches or data compromise have substantially reduced—indeed almost eliminated—over the years. This is in part because of the fact that technology has matured and also because customers have become used to following basic precautions necessary for safely using such services. Many financial institutions also offer their services via the Cloud. Customers can review their accounts, transfer funds and perform other operations over the web. Millions of customers avail of these services. The earlier apprehensions about the security of financial data hosted in the Cloud have largely dissipated and customers have begun to value the tremendous convenience of using these services.

The Healthcare industry is however different from most other industry verticals. Healthcare data is highly sensitive—any breach of privacy and security in context of healthcare data can have serious consequences. Secondly, there are multiple entities that have to deal with healthcare data. This includes care providers, hospital administration staff, payers, labs, patients themselves.

There are extensive regulations governing the healthcare industry and many of these regulations impact the nature of the Information technology solutions adopted by the industry. The fact that Cloud-based solutions are being reliably used in other industry segments does not automatically imply that they can be used in the healthcare industry.

4.1 HEALTHCARE IT IS DIFFERENT FROM IT USED IN OTHER INDUSTRIES

There are a few key differences between the Healthcare industry and other industries in which Cloud-based systems have been used.

4.1.1 High risk industry

The healthcare industry impacts individuals to a greater extent than any other industry. Errors in the medical industry can be far costlier than similar errors in other fields. A report by AHRQ (Agency for Healthcare Research and Quality) [1] stated that in the period 2000–2002, an average of 195,000 people died annually in the US due to medical errors. Although this number has substantially reduced since then, it still numbers in tens of thousands. Such errors are estimated to cost the US about $17 Billion annually [2]. It is therefore essential that all systems used in the healthcare industry are robust and reliable. This applies to IT systems used in healthcare as well.

4.1.2 Highly regulated

Numerous Federal and state regulations govern the administration of healthcare in the US. Many other countries in the world have similar regulations. These regulations not only govern the responsibilities and obligations of various players in the industry, but they also determine the nature, functionality, safeguards of the IT systems that are used by each of them. In the US, the Health Insurance Portability and Accountability Act (HIPAA) defines the privacy and security regulations that are to be implemented in the IT systems used by various Covered Entities (includes care providers—physicians, nurse practitioners, hospitals, clinics, payers, insurance companies, etc.). The American Recovery and Reinvestment Act (ARRA) defines modifications to the HIPAA, and additionally creates incentives/penalties for adopting/not adopting EMR solutions. In addition, mandated certifying authorities exist that certify the IT products and systems that can be used by Covered Entities.

Any IT system that is to be used in the Healthcare industry must therefore comply with the significant volume of regulation, and also obtain a certification demonstrating that it meets the requirement of regulations.

Another consequence of these substantial regulations is that Covered Entities perceive significant legal risks and therefore there is a natural reluctance to adopt products and technologies that are either 'new' or have not been established.

4.1.3 Multiple stakeholders

There are a large number of stakeholders in the healthcare industry. This includes the patients, the physicians, the nurse practitioners, the hospitals/clinics, their administrative staff members, the payers/ insurance companies, employers, pharmaceutical companies, technology vendors, device manufacturers, government bodies, and so on. Healthcare information often needs to pass from one of these entities to another. Therefore the healthcare industry has extensive standards for data and information exchange, and any IT system needs to comply with these standards. The Health Level 7 (HL7) is an example of such a standard.

4.1.4 Slow Pace of Adoption

The Healthcare industry has traditionally been slow to adopt IT, especially the smaller clinics and single physician practices. It is estimated [3] that in 2007, 2.3% of all medical practices used a fully functional EMR system, while 25% used some EMR system, although fully functional EMR systems have been available for decades. The installation of any new IT product is viewed as disruptive because it is typically accompanied by a significant period of training and loss of productivity in the short term.

4.1.5 Small and Large Providers

It is estimated that out of the approximately 650,000 physicians in the US, half the number are office based, working with smaller clinics or as individual practitioners. These practitioners typically do not have the resources (in house IT staff, time, etc.) to evaluate or experiment with new IT systems. On the other hand there are many large multi-specialty hospitals whose IT requirements are distinctly different from those of office practitioners. In many of the other industry verticals, it is the smaller companies which are at the forefront of adopting new IT offerings. This does not apply to healthcare IT.

4.1.6 Long Term Relationships

In many other industry verticals, it is not uncommon to change IT vendors and products from time to time. However, in healthcare, changing IT systems frequently is not easy and there is hence an expectation that any product adopted would be good to use for several years if not a decade.

Given all of these differences, it is not clear that Cloud-based systems would work as well in the Healthcare industry as they have in other industry verticals, unless Cloud-based healthcare solutions address these unique attributes of the industry.

4.2 CLOUD-BASED SYSTEMS FOR HEALTHCARE IT

In the previous section we discussed some of the unique characteristics of the healthcare industry. In this book we will focus on Healthcare IT solutions for office practitioners, small clinics, and single physician practices and those practices that cannot justify full-time in-house IT staff. This group forms a significant percentage of the healthcare provider industry. Many Cloud-based solutions are now available for this group of practitioners which address virtually every requirement of such a practice. From a functionality standpoint, Cloud-based systems provide capabilities on par with traditional on-site systems as we will see in this chapter.

In this chapter, we will review the different classes of Cloud-based solutions available for Healthcare IT. Rather than describing specific products, our objective is to review the type of functionality that is supported or delivered by commercial Cloud-based systems available today.

4.2.1 Cloud-based EMR Systems

The HITECH Act makes it virtually incumbent on all care providers to transition to a system of electronic medical records. There are financial incentives for doing so until 2015, and thereafter there are penalties (Medicare/Medicaid linked) for those who do not adopt Electronic Medical Records (EMR). From a clinical perspective, EMR leads to improvement in the quality of care provided to patients. Cloud-based EMRs are therefore a key component of any Cloud-based healthcare offering.

What is EMR?

An EMR (electronic medical record) is a computer-based documentation of a patient's medical history including illnesses, examinations, reports, diagnosis and the care administered. Electronic Medical Records are created and maintained by care providers (physicians, nurses, hospital or lab staff, etc.) when a patient avails service from the provider. EMRs are also called Electronic Health Records or Medical charts. Because the Electronic Medical Record contains the entire medical history of an individual, they are treated as private information and there are clear legal guidelines for their handling and storage.

[Note: EMR is distinct from PHR (Personal Health Records) which refer to the health records created and maintained by the patients themselves.]

An EMR gives the care provider a complete understanding of the patient's medical history, including previous surgeries or hospitalizations, illnesses, laboratory tests, treatments, as well as information about allergies, habits and immunizations. It therefore makes available to the care provider the correct and complete context within which the provider can plan and provide further care.

There is no single format for EMR; multiple standards have been defined and are in use. The nature of the information contained within an EMR may therefore vary slightly depending on the specialty of the practice and the EMR software used.

The following key pieces of medical information however, are a part of virtually all EMR systems:

4.2.1.1 Patient Identification information

This not only includes identifying information such as patient's name, address, contact information, social security number etc., but can also includes family information, race, religion, and such other social and demographic information.

4.2.1.2 Information about Patient Allergies and Habits

This includes information about patient habits that impact health such as usage of alcohol or tobacco, diet, exercise schedule, sexual orientation, and so on. It also includes information about allergies or reactions to specific drugs or medications. The allergy information is particularly useful because it helps physicians avoid prescribing medication that would have otherwise led to allergic reaction.

4.2.1.3 Immunization Record

The immunization record includes the history of vaccinations or reports of tests demonstrating immunity to particular illnesses.

4.2.1.4 Medical History

This includes a chronological record of all medical encounters of the patient. An 'encounter' can mean anything from a simple visit to a physician for a minor illness to an incident of hospitalization for a complex surgical procedure.

For each encounter listed, the information in the EMR usually includes the following:

1) Information about the primary complaint—which is the problem for which the patient is seeing the doctor. This includes information about the symptoms, the history of the complaint, i.e., how long the patient is suffering from the specific complaint or whether the patient has sought treatment for that complaint in the past.
2) Information about prior health of the patient, including any history of the same illness or symptoms.
3) Summary of the physician's observations resulting from a physical examination of different organs, vital signs, particularly those related to the symptoms reported by the patient. There is also a record of the physician's diagnosis and assessment of the ailment and plan for treatment, i.e., the further course of action and any instructions or orders provided by the physician to other healthcare personnel.

4) Dates and results of medical findings such as laboratory tests, diseases or illnesses. The results of testing include for example blood tests, radiology examinations such as X-rays, CT/MRI, pathology or biopsy tests and any other tests related to a particular specialty.

5) Details of surgery if any, including operative reports and narratives.

6) Details of hospitalization including daily updates of patient progress including clinical changes as observed by physicians, their assistants and nurses, consultation information entered by visiting specialists or a family physician.

7) Details of prescriptions and referrals.

8) Digitized images such as those from X-Ray scans can also be attached to the Electronic Medical Record.

In addition, the EMR also contains information that is specific to each particular specialty.

The EMR is updated after every medical encounter.

Benefits of EMR

There are significant advantages to using EMR when compared to the more traditional paper-based records and charts.

1) **Storage**. In most countries, there are regulations governing the preservation of medical records (In the US, this period is typically 7 years). Care Providers need to preserve all their records at least for this mandated time, although many providers actually retain their records for an even longer duration. Storing paper-based records not only requires a larger amount of storage space, but it is also cumbersome because it involves substantial human effort. Eventually this translates into a higher cost for storing (and retrieving) paper-based records. Records, when digitized and converted to electronic form, take far lesser storage space (per unit of information) and they are also much easier to search and retrieve.

2) **Usage in Emergency**. Paper records are usually stored at off-site locations, and are difficult to access quickly, for example in cases of emergency. In a situation where a patient needs earlier paper records at a location other than the clinic which created

them, they take a long time to be transported. Communicating electronic records over long distances is significantly easier and faster, and it can make a critical different when care has to be administered to a patient at short notice.

3) **Duplication and Transportation costs.** Paper records involve significant costs to duplicate (copy) and transport (mail/fax). Duplication and transportation of electronic records is virtually free.

4) **Uniformity.** It is harder to maintain uniformity within paper-based records and charts because it is harder to standardize codes, abbreviations, terminology and formats. Non-uniformly created records can contribute to medical errors, especially if they are written in a poorly legible manner.

5) **Risks.** Because paper records are harder to duplicate, transport and store, they run a higher risk of being destroyed either by error or by act of nature such as floods, hurricanes or fire. It is a fact that the areas affected by Hurricane Katrina saw a remarkably faster adoption of EMR after most of the older records were lost due to the hurricane.

6) **Audit/Reporting.** It is much easier to audit electronic records as opposed to paper-based records. Electronic records are easier to analyze for statistics or for the purpose of reporting to government agencies.

7) **Integration.** EMR systems are easier to integrate with other systems such as Practice Management systems, ePrescription systems or billing systems. Such integration eventually results in better care for the patient.

8) **Efficiency.** There are studies which claim that EMR enhances the efficiency of healthcare administration [4], [5], [6] although there are other studies that dispute such findings [7].

To summarize, Electronic Medical Records are uniform, are easier to create and maintain and can be communicated quickly to the point of administration of care. There are probably a few hundred different EMR systems today, which include numerous Cloud-based systems. Cloud-based EMR systems are available for most specialties such as Cardiology, Dermatology, Endocrinology, ENT/Otolaryngology, Family Practice, Gastroenterology, General Surgery, Internal Medicine, Neurology, OB-GYN, Ophthalmology,

Orthopedics, Pain Management, Pediatrics, Podiatry, Psychiatry, Pulmonology, Urology and many others. The nature of the data that is captured and stored in a Cloud-based EMR differs from one specialty to another.

Cloud-based EMR systems have all the features and capabilities of in house-EMR systems. Many Cloud-based systems have rich and extremely easy-to-use interfaces along with the ability to customize the fields in the records. Cloud-based EMR systems make it even easier to access or transfer medical information to any point, for example to the point of care in an emergency. Cloud-based EMR also makes it easier to provide access to the records to the patient via patient portals.

4.2.2 Cloud-based Practice Management

A Cloud-based medical practice management application enables a healthcare provider to manage and streamline practice management tasks and workflows. A 'workflow' is a sequence of steps followed in order to attain a specific objective. Provision of healthcare involves execution of several workflows within the practice, mirroring the movement of the patient within the system. For example, there are clinical workflows that have to do with administration of clinical care from the time an appointment is scheduled through the time the patient is checked out. Similarly, there are workflows that follow and maintain claim information from the time that the encounter is first entered into the system until the point that the claim is paid. Different practices have different workflows—i.e., each practice may follow a different sequence of steps, gather slightly different pieces of information at each step, and so on. Medical Practice Management relates to the management of various workflows within the practice. Medical Practice Management Systems are therefore the key to ensuring that all operations within the practice run smoothly and efficiently.

Practice Management software deployed by a large hospital naturally differs from that intended for office based practices because the workflows employed are different. Some clinics/hospitals have multiple locations, and the Practice Management software needs to ensure that these multiple sites can easily share information and can work together in an integrated fashion. Furthermore, the features in Practice Management software often depend on the specialty for which it is intended. Different specialties clearly have different requirements and this is reflected in the Practice Management solutions they use. Given all of the above, the ability to customize the software to reflect the needs of a specific practice is an important characteristic of good Practice Management software. Practice Management software also needs to integrate with other software modules used by providers such as software for Electronic Medical Records (EMR), Electronic Prescriptions, Documentation, Laboratory software, Ambulatory software and so on.

Cloud-based Practice Management software usually supports features such as:

1) Appointment scheduling of patients
2) Eligibility and authorization
3) Physician scheduling, scheduling surgery or other procedures for patients
4) Tracking patient referrals
5) Patient account management
6) Managing patients as they move from admission to discharge including information on hospital rounds
7) Managing patient recall
8) Claims submission and processing, automated follow-ups, collections and remittance advice
9) Managing the schedules of employees of the clinic
10) Managing the inventory of medical supplies and office materials
11) Inter and intra clinic/location communication
12) HIPAA compliance
13) Patient portal

Using Practice Management software usually leads to a more streamlined administration of healthcare.

Partly due to the new regulations in the US, single physician practices and small clinics are likely to see an increased cost of doing business at least for some time, until they create systems to efficiently meet the new reporting and compliance requirements.

Reimbursements however are likely to shrink over time. This puts pressure on the small practices to enhance efficiencies of their business and Practice Management software is a key to accomplishing this objective. If patient workflows are streamlined, it results in better usage of human resources within the practice, thereby allowing the physician to see more patients within the same amount of time. Good Practice Management software can positively impact the financial performance of a clinic or a physician practice. Practice management software also assists in the tracking of claims therefore leading to quicker reimbursements and better cash-flows.

There are several commercially available Cloud-based Practice Management solutions that support the requirements listed above. In a Cloud-based Practice Management solution, the software is accessed in a browser over the Internet, which is why continuous Internet availability is essential. Cloud-based Practice Management solutions can be customized, although admittedly to a limited extent when compared to on-site solutions. However, Cloud-based solutions can effectively compete with the on-site solutions in terms of functionality and features.

4.2.3 Patient Portals

Healthcare regulation makes it mandatory for all EMR systems to provide a Patient Portal. A patient portal is essentially a website on which patients can log in and access most portions of their medical records.

From a technology stand-point, the patient portal is a front end that interacts with the healthcare IT system of the healthcare provider, and can access the data stored there. The data-views (screens/dialogs in which the data is displayed) are obviously different for physicians and patients, although the data displayed is accessed from the same database. In a patient portal, the information is presented in a manner which makes it easy for the patient (a layman) to understand the nature of his conditions and his treatment. In an EMR system (used by physicians/nurse practitioners), the data is presented in a manner that is appropriate for trained medical personnel. Most patient portals do not communicate certain types of highly sensitive information, such as treatment for HIV/AIDS or addiction treatment.

Most Patient Portals also provide for some level of interactivity with the healthcare provider. For example, they provide capability allowing patients to:

1) Schedule new appointments or modify previously scheduled appointments with the care provider
2) Register or complete any forms (including medical history) online (thereby saving time at the clinic)
3) Send messages to physicians or ask questions
4) Request prescription medication refills
5) Review billing information and make payments online
6) Review further educational information pertaining to their condition.

In addition, Patient Portals serve the following important functions:

1) They help the patient understand the nature of his ailment, the diagnosis and the course of treatment. Patients can use this information to find out more information about their condition from other sources such as the Internet and better participate in the treatment.
2) Patients can obtain second-opinions from other physicians on the course of the treatment based on the information available in the patient portal. The portal saves them the effort of actually seeking out their medical information from their primary care provider.
3) In situations where a patient seeks care at a location other than their primary care provider, and access to prior medical records is essential, the patient portal provides a convenient way to quickly access prior medical records.

[Note: Patient Portals reflect information generated by the healthcare provider. They are therefore different from Personal Health Records (PHR) systems—which are self-help websites on which patients can maintain their own medical information/records for their own use.]

Patient Portals represent one of the key advantages of Cloud-based systems over in-house systems. A Patient Portal interfaces with sensitive, private information of individuals and they need to be securely available and web-accessible at all times. It is therefore best if the responsibility of managing the patient portal is assigned to an entity that has the know-how, the infrastructure, the resources and the experience to design and manage high availability, high security information systems. Most clinics or physician practices do not have this capability, nor is it practically feasible to invest in infrastructure and human resources in order to guarantee such capability. It is therefore best to opt for a Patient Portal that is Cloud-based. Since the patient Portal accesses the same data as an EMR/Patient Management system, it ends up being beneficial to use a Cloud-based EMR system as well.

4.2.4 Cloud-based ePrescription

Many Practice Management systems and EMR systems include ePrescription capability as a part of their overall functionality. However, because ePrescription is so important, and there are standalone systems for ePrescription, we will cover these systems separately in this section. ePrescription is also one of the criteria mentioned in the definition of 'meaningful use' in HITECH Act.

Traditionally, a large percentage of the prescriptions created annually in the US (totally numbering to a few billion) have been handwritten by physicians or nurse practitioners. Hand written prescriptions are often illegible and this results in a large number of medication errors. When prescriptions are not legible, they are often followed by phone calls/callbacks made from pharmacies to physicians because of the pharmacy's inability to understand the prescriptions. In the worst case, hand written prescriptions that are not legible can result in wrong medicines being provided to the patient. When prescriptions are written by hand, patients need to approach their physicians every time they need to refill their medication.

An ePrescription system is a computerized system in which the prescription is either entered by the physician/nurse practitioner or generated on the basis of data available to the system. The prescription can be automatically communicated to pharmacies associated with the healthcare provider. Further, ePrescription systems also have inbuilt rules/databases pertaining to drug-drug allergies and appropriateness of each drug in the context of various health conditions. Thus, the system automatically ensures that a specific prescription does not lead to drug-drug allergies and that a drug does not lead to negative effects based on all the medical information about the patient available in the system.

ePrescription systems are an excellent example of how IT can have measurably beneficial impact in the administration of healthcare. An ePrescription system brings several benefits:

1) It eliminates the possibility of a prescription being incorrectly interpreted due to bad handwriting, thereby reducing medical errors. It eliminates the necessity for follow-up phone calls or faxes from pharmacies to physicians which happen when a prescription is not clearly legible. This saves physicians and nurses a substantial amount of time. According to a survey conducted by Medco Health Solutions, Inc. in 2003 of Boston area physicians [8], 88 percent of those surveyed said that roughly a third of the time of medical staff is spent responding to phone calls from pharmacies regarding prescriptions.

2) It reduces the instance of drug-drug allergies and the possibility of inappropriate drug being administered in the view of the patients overall medical history.

3) It makes ordering refills easier, since prior prescriptions can be easily accessed electronically.

4) ePrescriptions are also found to enhance compliance by patients simply because they are more convenient.

As we saw earlier, the ability of small clinics and office based physicians to maintain high uptimes with their IT systems cannot match that of Cloud service providers. Consequently, a Cloud-based ePrescription system is likely to be much more highly available and secure and therefore be able to communicate prescriptions to pharmacies with higher reliability than an in-house system. Secondly, a Cloud-based system is more likely to collaborate with more and more pharmacy chains over a period of time, enhancing the number of pharmacies your ePrescriptions can be sent to.

There are several Cloud-based ePrescription systems that are available either as stand-alone systems or as a part of comprehensive Cloud-based healthcare IT solutions.

4.2.5 Online storage of Data and Images, Online Backups

Healthcare IT systems generate a large volume of data on a daily basis. The data storage system on which this data is stored is referred to as primary storage. There are several reasons why the data on the primary storage needs to be backed up (i.e., replicated and archived) on secondary storage. These include loss or corruption of data on primary storage due to failure of hardware or software, virus infections, electrical outages or power surges resulting in corruption of data, fire, theft, vandalism, floods, hurricanes or other acts of nature, data being destroyed due to human error, etc. It is best if the secondary storage is physically remote from the primary

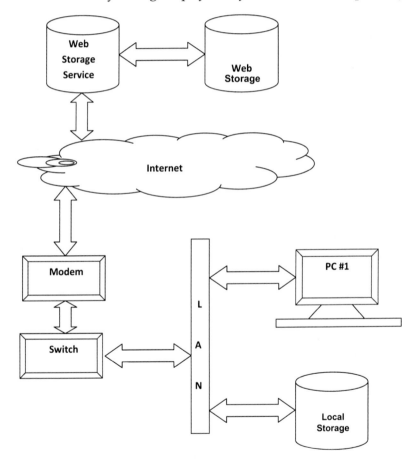

Fig 4.1 Schematic of Cloud-based storage. A client software running on PC #1 can continuously backup data on Local Storage to Web-based storage.

storage location. Many physician practices with in-house IT backup their data daily on tapes/USB storage and an administrator carries the storage device home.

Even if your clinic/practice does not use Cloud-based systems for practice management, EMR, etc., it is a good idea to consider Cloud-based systems for data backup and secondary storage. The way most Cloud-based backup systems work is as follows:

There is software installed on one or more of the computers within your facility (called the backup client) connected to your primary storage. In case of certain Cloud-based systems, this software runs in a web-browser window rather than running natively. The backup client tracks the changes to the data stored on the primary storage at regular intervals and communicates the changes to the Cloud-based storage facility of the service provider. This assumes that an internet connection is available at all times. In this way, the data on the primary storage within your clinic is periodically replicated on the remote Cloud-based storage. The Cloud backup provider has a copy of all your data at all times. You can access this copy should anything go wrong with your primary data storage. In many systems, it is also possible to roll back and obtain from the Cloud provider a snapshot of your data at an earlier point in time. (Provision for such capability naturally increases the overall storage requirement, but is very useful from the perspective of an audit, should the need arise).

The backup client encrypts all data before it is communicated to Cloud storage. Secondly, bandwidth requirements are substantially reduced because the client only communicates the changes that have occurred in the data since the last backup cycle, rather than transmitting all the data again. Figure 4.1 shows a schematic of a remote backup mechanism.

There are clear HIPAA guidelines for storage and transmission of healthcare data. These guidelines include a combination of administrative controls and technical safeguards for data transmission and storage as we will see in a subsequent chapter.

Examples of administrative controls include:

1) Physical protection of locations where data is stored
2) Automation and audit trails of backup process

3) Long-term (up to 7 years) of data storage
4) Controls on who has access to data
5) Procedures and guidelines for Breach notification

Examples of Technical safeguards include:

1) Encryption of data (minimum key sizes and acceptable protocols are defined) while in transit from one place to another
2) Encryption of stored data
3) Controls on access to encryption passwords.

There are several commercially available cloud backup products which conform to these guidelines.

When you sign up with a Cloud-based backup provider, it is important to at least once go through the process of complete data recovery from the backup. This is done in the following steps:

1) Backup all the data on your primary storage on a tape drive.
2) Clean (i.e., erase) all the data on your primary storage to mimic a situation involving complete loss of data.
3) Obtain a latest image of all your data from your Cloud-based backup provider.
4) Install the data image obtained from your Cloud provider back onto your primary storage.
5) Verify that no data has been lost and that the system continues to work as it should.

The verification that there is no data loss can be done with one of several commercially available tools. One idea underlying these tools involves taking a cryptographic hash of all your data on primary storage initially, and then comparing it with the cryptographic hash of the data after you have recovered it from the Cloud provider. There are also standard tools available to compare data in two files that can be used to make the comparison.

The purpose of going through this exercise at least once is to ensure that you can indeed bring up your systems based on the backup residing at the Cloud provider. In case of an actual fire/theft incident, this process would need to be replicated (but without the safety of the tape drive backup of step 1).

When all your systems are Cloud-based, you do not have to worry about issues such as remote backup and recovery. Most Cloud providers have a system for backing up all their data remotely. (You need to verify this when you sign up with a Cloud-based vendor.) They also establish processes to ensure rapid and accurate recovery of data from their backup systems. This means that your data is always available to you when you need it.

An important special case of a data backup system is the Picture Archival and Communication System ('PACS'). In the process of administering healthcare, numerous images, graphs, pictures and scans are generated—information that has to be stored pictorially rather than in a textual form. This includes for example images from X-Rays, Ultrasound machines, MRI and CT scans, endoscopy, mammograms, computed radiography, etc. Even scanned images of paper documents are often required to be stored, for example, when legacy paper-based information is digitized via scanning. In order to ensure uniformity, a standard format used to store and communicate pictorial information has been defined—the Digital Imaging and Communications in Medicine ('DICOM').

Several Cloud-based PACS systems are commercially available today. In these systems, as described earlier, the client software modules run on primary storage devices. *[Note: Earlier in this section we assumed there was a single primary storage device. It is also possible that there are multiple primary storage devices on the internal network of the clinic—for example the primary storage could be the individual computers or capture devices that are on the LAN.]* There is a server in the cloud with which the individual client modules communicate. This server has an image database and the ability to store actual images. Images from any of the computers or capture devices can be backed up to the server via the client software modules. Similarly, any image stored on the cloud server can be retrieved using the client software module or via a standard browser.

Browser based viewers can incorporate all the functionality including advanced visualization capability and analysis capability that native image viewers provide.

Cloud-based backup for data and images is something that healthcare providers should consider, even if their EMR systems are not Cloud-based.

4.2.6 Departmental Solutions: Laboratory, Radiology

Unlike large multi-specialty hospitals, most clinics and physician practices do not have in-house Laboratory or Radiology setups. They therefore often refer patients to stand-alone Laboratory/ Radiology centers. These centers are an important link in the administration of care to patients. There are several Cloud-based IT solutions tailored for Laboratories, Radiology centers, and other such Testing facilities. These solutions are collectively referred to as Departmental Solutions.

Laboratories and Radiology Centers are low margin businesses. They are subject to extensive regulations as well. There is hence a push to process an ever larger number of patients in order to enhance revenues. The goal of Departmental IT Solutions is to enhance efficiency, reduce costs, ensure compliance and improve quality of care by improving the decision making and reporting functions. Many of these systems also include advanced analytic and reporting tools.

Cloud-based Laboratory solutions are available for various functions such as Microbiology, histology and cytology processes, Synoptic/Antibiogram reporting, Image/Document capture, Inventory Management, Voice recording, Blood bank, etc. They have all the functionality of on-site solutions.

Cloud-based Radiology systems are similar to PACS systems discussed in the earlier section. These systems support basic Radiology workflows where physicians can register examination requests for existing or new patients, and select appropriate billing rules. The technician can upload the radiology images and link them to the specific examination request for that patient. Finally the radiologist can review the images and create reports. All of these functions are handled inside a web-browser, and there is no need to install any software on any computer.

It is also possible to interface laboratory devices directly to Cloud-based systems. This means that the readings from instruments or captured images are directly uploaded to the cloud. Such functionality however does require the presence of 'driver software' or 'plug-ins' that runs natively on the computer connected to the measuring /imaging device.

4.2.7 Mobility Solutions

Mobile healthcare solutions are popular among medical professionals who are unlikely to be at their desk all the time. Mobile healthcare solutions are IT solutions that run on hand-held devices, such as mobile phones, tablets, or other specialized hardware that is easy for physicians and nurse practitioners to carry. Any handheld device which has an Internet Browser can be used to access a Cloud-based solution. In other words, one does not need a desktop or laptop computer to access Cloud-based solutions. There is a great deal of convenience for a physician to be able to look up the details/status of a patient from home or on the road.

There are other mobile solutions in addition to devices with browsers that are capable of accessing standard Cloud-based offerings. Many vendors offer customized hardware solutions tailored to the Healthcare industry. For example, there are handheld devices which interface with other devices such as glucometers or blood-pressure measuring instruments over wireless communication in order to obtain the readings. There are handheld devices that directly authenticate patient's wristbands and smart cards to pull up the patient's information.

Another important class of applications on mobile platforms are voice-based applications. Some of these applications are:

1) Being able to record voice segments into a mobile/handheld device and store them in the Cloud.
2) Ability to dictate medical notes/emails/etc. into a handheld device and access them later.
3) Run a search on the stored information (e.g. EMR system) using a voice-command and search phrase.

Some of these systems are Cloud-based and all data resides in the Datacenter.

4.3 ADVANTAGES OF CLOUD-BASED HEALTHCARE IT SYSTEMS

In earlier chapters, we discussed in general the advantages and disadvantages of Cloud-based systems vis-à-vis in-house systems.

In this section we will review these advantages/disadvantages specifically in the context of healthcare systems.

4.3.1 Cloud-based solutions are Cost effective

Cloud-based solutions are distinctly cost effective when compared to on-site solutions. Here, cost comparison is based on total costs associated with using a particular solution which includes the costs of hardware, software, personnel, infrastructure, etc. on one hand, and the monthly subscription fees on the other.

4.3.2 Convenience

Particularly for smaller clinics and independent physician practices, using Cloud-based systems is more convenient. Your practice does not have to worry about backups, security of data or ensuring that your systems/patient portals are available 24x7.

4.3.3 Collaboration and Mobility

Cloud-based systems allow physicians to collaborate on any medical data easily and also allow physicians to access and work on the system from anywhere, including from home.

4.3.4 Patient Portal, ePrescribing

Providing these functions require physicians to provide 24x7 external access to healthcare systems. This is best done with a Cloud-based system.

4.3.5 Easier to get started

The process of evaluating a Cloud-based systems is typically faster and adoption is easier. This also has to do with the fact that the upfront investment is smaller.

4.4 ASP MODELS AND CLOUD-BASED SYSTEMS

Many healthcare IT providers provide an ASP-type option to their customers. The ASP option has the following characteristics:

1) The IT system instead of residing on computers within the clinic/physician practice, resides on servers at a Datacenter under the control of the software vendor.

2) The software is accessed from the clinic using a technology such as Virtual Private network (VPN) or other similar technologies for remote access. (e.g. Citrix). This means that the computers within the clinic need to have the VPN/remote access client installed on them.

3) The software vendor typically sets aside a number of physical servers for your use, and installs a version of his systems on these servers. These servers and the system running on them are for your dedicated use. If your requirements are small, the vendor may partition a single physical server into multiple logical servers and assign you one of these logical servers. This is different from the 'multi-tenancy' model adopted by Cloud-providers, and is in the category of 'virtualization'.

4) The software vendor is responsible for regular upgrades to your system, and also for ensuring that your servers are up and accessible at all times. The vendor is also responsible for data backups.

5) The software vendor bills you on a 'pay-as-you-go' basis, i.e., you pay typically monthly commensurate with your level of usage.

There is no significant difference from a customer perspective, in the ASP model and the Cloud model. In both cases, the software is remotely hosted and accessed over the internet. The vendor is responsible for software and server maintenance, ensuring system uptime and data backups. In both cases, there is no upfront capital cost and you pay for using the software as a service. The only difference pertains to using the browser in one case and using a VPN software in case of ASP. This also means that ASP type solutions may not be accessible from hand-held devices that cannot run a VPN, whereas Cloud solutions are.

Most on-site solution vendors now offer their solutions as a service via this ASP model. This has increased the choice of IT solutions available to clinics and physicians.

4.5 SUMMARY

To summarize, Cloud-based solutions available for clinical and non-clinical tasks include all the functionality of in-house systems. They are cost-effective, and easy to get started with.

REFERENCES

[1] http://www.medicalnewstoday.com/articles/11856.php

[2] http://www.ahrq.gov/qual/errback.htm

[3] *National Health Statistic Report*, No. 23, 2010, Esther Hing, M.P.H., and Chun-Ju Hsiao, Ph.D., Division of Health Care Statistics

[4] http://www.thedigitalclinic.com/imgs/pdfs/OrthoPad%20Case%20Study_TOC.pdf

[5] https://www.ncbi.nlm.nih.gov/pmc/articles/PMC1839545/

[6] http://www.eurekalert.org/pub_releases/2008-11/hms-ehr112508.php

[7] *Hospital Computing and the Costs and Quality of Care: A National Study*, David U. Himmelstein, Adam Wright, Steffie Woolhandler, American Journal of Medicine, 2009.

[8] http://www.hoise.com/vmw/03/articles/vmw/LV-VM-03-03-25.html

CHAPTER 5

HIPAA and HITECH—Cloud Perspective

Conforming to applicable laws and regulations is the foremost concern of any medical practitioner. There are Federal as well as State regulations in addition to guidelines issued by applicable practice boards. The key federal regulations dealing with Information Technology in Healthcare are the HIPAA (Health Insurance Portability & Accountability Act) and the subsequent amendments to it contained in the HITECH Act (The Health Information Technology for Economic and Clinical Health Act). The HITECH Act also provides incentives for practices to adopt and demonstrate "meaningful use" of Electronic Health Records. Many practitioners question whether the use of Cloud-based services conforms to the provisions of HIPAA & HITECH and whether such use qualifies their practices for financial incentives under the HITECH Act. In this chapter we will review some of the key aspects of applicable regulations and the obligations they impose upon healthcare providers. We will evaluate whether these obligations can be fulfilled by practices using Cloud-based services and how easy or hard it is to do so.

This chapter is not intended to be a substitute for legal advice. Our intention is to only provide an overview of some of the regulations in the context of Cloud-based solutions.

5.1 WHAT IS HIPAA

The Health Insurance Portability & Accountability Act of 1996 (HIPAA), a US Federal Law, became effective in July 1997. The objectives of this act were:

1) To combat waste, fraud, abuse; to reduce costs and enhance the overall efficiency and effectiveness of healthcare delivery and insurance industry.
2) To enhance the ability of various entities in the healthcare industry to exchange information via standardization.
3) To ensure the confidentiality and security of personal health information.
4) To ensure portability and continuity of health insurance coverage.

HIPAA simplifies the administration of health insurance, makes it easier to access long term healthcare services and protects health coverage of individuals and families when they transition jobs. It limits exclusions based on pre-existing conditions and prohibits discrimination against workers on the basis of their health status. It also allows the portability of group coverage between two carriers.

HIPAA's provisions apply to

1) Health Plans
2) Health Care Providers
3) Health Care Clearinghouses

The term 'Healthcare Providers' includes single physician or multi-physician practices, clinics, hospitals, etc. The text of the Act can be downloaded from [1] or [2] and detailed commentaries on this act are available at [3], [4].

While the Act deals extensively with issues relating insurance coverage, the Administrative Simplification procedures contained in the Act directly pertain to the Information Technology Infrastructure, polices and processes utilized and followed by the Health Care Provider.

5.1.1 HIPAA Administrative Simplification

In line with its stated objective to promote efficiency in the administration of healthcare, HIPAA includes 'Administrative Simplifications' which, as the name suggests, are intended to simplify the processes and information management procedures related to healthcare. The most effective way to bring about process simplification is by enhancing the use of Information Technology.

Greater computerization typically reduces overall costs by minimizing or even eliminating paperwork which in turn leads to lesser administrative overheads on medical staff. This is what the HIPAA Administrative Simplification seeks to do. To quote from the Act:

> "It is the purpose of this subtitle to improve the Medicare program under title XVIII of the Social Security Act, the Medicaid program under title XIX of such Act, and the efficiency and effectiveness of the health care system, by encouraging the development of a health information system through the establishment of standards and requirements for the electronic transmission of certain health information."

Administrative Simplification has been proposed with the objective of making business practice (the billing, claims, computer systems and communication) uniform. These simplifications affect activities such as:

1) Enrolling an individual in a health plan
2) Paying health insurance premiums
3) Checking eligibility
4) Obtaining authorization to refer a patient to a specialist
5) Processing claims
6) Notifying a provider about the payment of a claim

With greater computerization and use of Information Technology however come the risks that are associated with data in an electronic form. Because Healthcare IT deals with sensitive, medical information, the Administrative Simplification in HIPAA also specifies the nature of precautions to be taken and processes to be followed for ensuring the privacy and security of healthcare data.

HIPAA authorizes the secretary of Health and Human Services (HHS) to define a common set of standards for electronic data interchange (EDI) in order to reduce the administrative costs associated with healthcare operations. Standardization of electronic formats for healthcare-related transactions includes creation of uniform code sets for clinical and non-clinical data exchange, unique identifiers for patients and providers, common transaction message formats, guidelines for ensuring security and privacy of healthcare information, and so on [5].

5.1.1.1 Standardization of Code Sets and Transaction Formats

The Transactions and Code Sets (TCS) Standard applies to all Covered entities and has been in effect since October 2003. It mandates uniform electronic exchange formats for all Covered Entities.

To quote from HIPAA, "the lack of common, industry-wide standards [is] a major obstacle to realizing potential efficiency and savings." Each insurer has a different format and procedure for filing health claims. Different providers have different forms for referrals and authorizations. Medical personnel and staff have to spend inordinate amount of time on administrative matters such as filling out forms, verifying eligibility and filing claims. As per estimates provided by [5], around 20 percent of health care costs are due to the paperwork involved. Significant efficiencies can be achieved if all transactions and communication between various healthcare entities are compliant with a common standard. Not only would this allow computers to process the information, but also significantly reduce human-errors in interpretation. Presently, standards are defined for the following types of common transactions:

1) claims payment and remittance advice
2) coordination of benefits
3) eligibility for a health plan
4) enrollment and disenrollment in a health plan
5) health care claim status
6) premium payments
7) referral certification and authorization.

Several organizations have already developed EDI standards for healthcare industry, and the Department of Health and Human Services (DHHS) has selected its standards from among those available. These include, at this time: Health Care Claims or equivalent encounter information (ANSI X12N 837), Eligibility for a Health Plan (ANSI X12N 270/271), Referral Certification and Authorization (ANSI X12N 278), Health Care Claim Status (ANSI X12N 276/277), Enrollment and Disenrollment in a Health Plan (ANSI X12N 834), Health Care Payment and Remittance Advice (ANSI X12N 835). However, the DHHS may modify or change the standards as appropriate via the formal rule-making process.

DHHS also defines a common set of codes that must be used for any electronic transaction. Presently, there are a number of codes that private and public entities use for their transactions. There are codes for specialized services offered by individual providers. It is necessary to have a common set of codes that are to be used by all entities. Such a common code set enhances efficiency by aiding computerization. DHHS has adopted a number of available code sets including

1) International Classification of Disease, Clinical Modification (ICD-CM)
2) National Drug Codes (NDC)
3) Code on Dental Procedures and Nomenclature (CDT)
4) Healthcare Common Procedure Coding System (HCPCS)
5) Current Procedure Terminology (CPT).

5.1.1.2 Standardized identifiers

As per HIPAA, the establishment of a unique identification scheme based on identification numbers can aid in quality improvement and reduction of costs. Each Covered Entity including providers, health plans, payers, employers, etc. is assigned a unique identification number using which the particular entity can be identified. This helps the faster processing of claims and because this identification number is to be quoted in all transactions and claims.

5.1.1.3 Privacy and security standards

All Covered Entities must adhere to a set of Privacy and Security standards while dealing with healthcare information. These standards place significant obligations on healthcare providers, and are discussed in detail in subsequent sections.

5.2 THE HITECH ACT

The HITECH Act i.e., The Health Information Technology for Economic and Clinical Health Act is part of the American Recovery and Reinvestment Act of 2009 (ARRA). The HITECH Act is intended to encourage more effective and efficient health care through the use of technology, thereby reducing the total cost of health care for all Americans and then using these savings to enable all Americans to have access to the health care system. Savings are expected to come from efficiency gains and improved clinical guidelines, allowing treatments to be standardized for various medical conditions. There are substantial incentives for the adoption of healthcare information technology in general, including the creation of a national healthcare infrastructure and the adoption of electronic health record (EHR) systems among providers. The purpose of this Act has been stated as follows [6].

(b) PURPOSE—The National Coordinator shall perform the duties under subsection (c) in a manner consistent with the development of a nationwide health information technology infrastructure that allows for the electronic use and exchange of information and that—

"1) ensures that each patient's health information is secure and protected, in accordance with applicable law;

"2) improves health care quality, reduces medical errors, reduces health disparities, and advances the delivery of patientcentered medical care;

"3) reduces health care costs resulting from inefficiency, medical errors, inappropriate care, duplicative care, and incomplete information;

"4) provides appropriate information to help guide medical decisions at the time and place of care;

"5) ensures the inclusion of meaningful public input in such development of such infrastructure;

"6) improves the coordination of care and information among hospitals, laboratories, physician offices, and other entities through an effective infrastructure for the secure and authorized exchange of health care information;

"7) improves public health activities and facilitates the early identification and rapid response to public health threats and emergencies, including bioterror events and infectious disease outbreaks;

"8) facilitates health and clinical research and health care quality;

"9) promotes early detection, prevention, and management of chronic diseases;

"10) promotes a more effective marketplace, greater competition, greater systems analysis, increased consumer choice, and improved outcomes in health care services; and

"11) improves efforts to reduce health disparities."

The HITECH Act anticipates a many-fold increase in the electronic storage and transfer of healthcare information. It therefore modifies the security and privacy provisions contained within HIPAA, and significantly broadens the scope, rigor and enforcement of those provisions. It increases the potential legal liability for non-compliance; and it provides for more enforcement.

The data privacy and security provisions of HIPAA are extended to Business Associates of healthcare providers, clinics, laboratories, pharmacies, etc. Business Associates are now also subject to penalties for breach of HIPAA provisions. The HITECH Act also substantially enhances the reporting requirements of providers and their Business Associates.

The HITECH Act provides financial incentives under Medicare/Medicaid for those providers who demonstrate 'meaningful use' of Electronic Health Records. The key components of 'meaningful use' include use of ePrescriptions, electronic exchange of PHI among systems and ability to meet clinical and non-clinical quality metrics. The HITECH Act provides significant financial incentives to healthcare providers for meeting the meaningful use guidelines for EHR adoption.

5.3 DEFINITIONS

In this section, we will list a few key definitions relevant to HIPAA and HITECH Acts.

5.3.1 Health Care Provider

The term 'health care provider' includes a hospital, skilled nursing facility, home health entity or other long term care facility, health care clinic, community mental health center (as defined in section 1913(b)(1)), renal dialysis facility, blood center, ambulatory surgical center described in section 1833(i) of the Social Security Act, emergency medical services provider, Federally qualified health center, group practice, a pharmacist, a pharmacy, a laboratory, a physician (as defined in section 1861(r) of the Social Security Act), a practitioner (as described in section 1842(b)(18)(C) of the Social Security Act), a provider operated by, or under contract with, the Indian Health Service or by an Indian tribe (as defined in the Indian Self-Determination and Education Assistance Act), tribal organization, or urban Indian organization (as defined in section 4 of the Indian Health Care Improvement Act), a rural health clinic, a Covered Entity under section 340B, an ambulatory surgical center described in section 1833(i) of the Social Security Act, a therapist (as defined in section 1848(k)(3)(B)(iii) of the Social Security Act), and any other category of health care facility, entity, 42 USC 300jj practitioner, or clinician determined appropriate by the Secretary.

5.3.2 Covered Entity or CE [Code of Federal Regulations—Title 45]

Covered entity means either of the following:

1) A health plan.
2) A health care clearinghouse.
3) A health care provider who transmits any health information in electronic form in connection with a transaction covered by this subchapter.

5.3.3 Health Information Technology

The term 'health information technology' means hardware, software, integrated technologies or related licenses, intellectual property, upgrades, or packaged solutions sold as services that are designed for or support the use by health care entities or patients for the electronic creation, maintenance, access, or exchange of health information.

5.3.4 Qualified Electronic Health Record

The term 'qualified electronic health record' means an electronic record of health-related information on an individual that

1) includes patient demographic and clinical health information, such as medical history and problem lists
2) has the capacity:
   i. to provide clinical decision support
   ii. to support physician order entry

    iii. to capture and query information relevant to health care quality

    iv. to exchange electronic health information with, and integrate such information from other sources

5.3.5 Certified Electronic Health Records

"The term 'certified EHR technology' means a qualified electronic health record that is certified pursuant to section 3001(c)(5) as meeting standards adopted under section 3004 that are applicable to the type of record involved (as determined by the Secretary, such as an ambulatory electronic health record for office-based physicians or an inpatient hospital electronic health record for hospitals)."

3001(c) (5) is as below:

CERTIFICATION

"(A) IN GENERAL.—The National Coordinator, in consultation with the Director of the National Institute of Standards and Technology, shall keep or recognize a program or programs for the voluntary certification of health information technology as being in compliance with applicable certification criteria adopted under this subtitle. Such program shall include, as appropriate, testing of the technology in accordance with section 13201(b) of the Health Information Technology for Economic and Clinical Health Act.

"(B) CERTIFICATION CRITERIA DESCRIBED.—In this title, the term 'certification criteria' means, with respect to standards and implementation specifications for health information technology, criteria to establish that the technology meets such standards and implementation specifications.

Section 3004, titled "PROCESS FOR ADOPTION OF ENDORSED RECOMMENDATIONS; ADOPTION OF INITIAL SET OF STANDARDS, IMPLEMENTATION SPECIFICATIONS, AND CERTIFICATION CRITERIA" states that the Secretary, HHS in consultation with representatives of other relevant Federal agencies, shall jointly review standards, implementation specifications, or certification criteria, and,

shall determine whether or not to propose adoption of such standards, implementation specifications, or certification criteria. It further states that the Secretary, HHS shall, through a rulemaking process, adopt an initial set of standards, implementation specifications, and certification criteria and that these may be issued on an interim, final basis.

In other words, the HITECH act specifies that Healthcare providers should adopt Certified EHR solutions, while responsibility of defining the certification criteria and process is with the Secretary, HHS.

From the perspective of providers who are looking to adopt EHR solutions, ensuring that the solution (whether it is a Cloud-based solution or an in-house solution) is certified as per HITECH guidelines is the first step in the selection process.

The rules, criteria and process for product certification are discussed in a later chapter.

5.3.6 Protected Health Information

Protected health information (PHI) under HIPAA includes any individually identifiable health information. This not only means information that can be explicitly linked to a particular individual, but also information that can 'reasonably allow' individual identification.

De-indentified information is one from which all identifying information (or potentially identifying information) has been removed.

Health Information itself has been defined as any information, whether oral or recorded in any form or medium that is created or received by a health care provider, health plan, public health authority, employer, life insurer, school or university, or health care clearinghouse and which relates to the past, present, or future physical or mental health or condition of an individual; the provision of health care to an individual; or the past, present, or future payment for the provision of health care to an individual.

All patient-related information that a healthcare provider deals with, is therefore covered under Protected Health Information, unless it is entirely de-identified.

5.3.7 Business Associate

The concept of 'Business Associate' is important to understand for healthcare providers. The definition of a Business Associate as per Code of Federal Regulations—Title 45 is as follows:

1) Except as provided in paragraph (2) of this definition, business associate means, with respect to a Covered Entity, a person who: (i) On behalf of such Covered Entity or of an organized health care arrangement (as defined in 164.501 of this subchapter) in which the Covered Entity participates, but other than in the capacity of a member of the workforce of such Covered Entity or arrangement, performs, or assists in the performance of: (A) A function or activity involving the use or disclosure of individually identifiable health information, including claims processing or administration, data analysis, processing or administration, utilization review, quality assurance, billing, benefit management, practice management, and repricing; or (B) Any other function or activity regulated by this subchapter; or (ii) Provides, other than in the capacity of a member of the workforce of such Covered Entity, legal, actuarial, accounting, consulting, data aggregation (as defined in 164.501 of this subchapter), management, administrative, accreditation, or financial services to or for such Covered Entity, or to or for an organized health care arrangement in which the Covered Entity participates, where the provision of the service involves the disclosure of individually identifiable health information from such Covered Entity or arrangement, or from another business associate of such Covered Entity or arrangement, to the person.

2) A Covered Entity participating in an organized health care arrangement that performs a function or activity as described by paragraph (1)(i) of this definition for or on behalf of such organized health care arrangement, or that provides a service as described in paragraph (1)(ii) of this definition to or for such organized health care arrangement, does not, simply through the performance of such function or activity or the

provision of such service, become a business associate of other Covered Entities participating in such organized health care arrangement.

3) A Covered Entity may be a business associate of another Covered Entity.

In other words, a Business Associate can be either an individual (not an employee of the Healthcare Provider) or a corporate entity that acts on behalf of the Healthcare provider and is engaged in activity that deals with health information in custody of the Healthcare Provider. So, for example, if you—the healthcare provider engage the services of a consultant or a vendor to perform any sort of data processing, administrative, accounting, legal, financial or any such function that gives them access to health information or medical records, these providers come under the definition of 'Business Associates'.

If you were to utilize a Cloud-based service for healthcare IT, the data processing and data storage would be performed by the Cloud provider. As per the above definition therefore, a provider of Cloud-based solutions should be considered a Business Associate and needs to assume the obligations of Business Associates as outlined in HIPAA and HITECH Act.

It is necessary for Healthcare Providers to enter into contracts with each of their Business Associates. These are known as Business Associate Contracts. Such a contract outlines the details of the activities that the Business Associate is authorized to perform on behalf of the Provider. Some of the important provisions contained within a Business Associate Contract include:

1) The provision that the information will be subject to appropriate physical and technical safeguards and shall be protected from unauthorized use or disclosure.

2) The provision that the Business Associate shall inform the provider and the appropriate government agencies of any breach of security or unauthorized use/disclosure of information as soon as the Business Associate becomes aware of it.

3) The provision that the obligations, restrictions and conditions of the Business Associate shall apply to all employees, agents, contractors, etc who have access to the information.

4) The provision that all information will be returned or destroyed upon termination of contract.

5) The provision that the Business Associate will work with the Provider to make relevant information available to the Patient (the patient who is the subject of that information).

6) The provision that the Business Associate will ensure compliance with all regulations and make available their internal books, processes, documents etc available for audit by any government agency.

Sample texts of contracts with Business Associates are available at [7] and [8]. These are intended to provide an overview of the nature of these contracts and may need to be modified depending on the nature of your relationship with a Business Associate. A sample contract is also provided in the Appendices.

When such a contract is entered into, healthcare providers are permitted to disclose protected health information to their Business Associates. Furthermore, those Business Associates are permitted to create, receive and manage such information on behalf of the provider.

The above provisions permit Providers to subscribe to Cloud-based solutions after entering into suitable Business Associate contracts with the Cloud providers. The provisions also allow the Cloud-provider to setup web-based portals for secure patient access to their data. Of course, it requires the Cloud provider to ensure that all data is suitably secured either in transit or while it is archived and stored.

As per DHHS, a Provider is not responsible or liable for violations of the Business Associate (Cloud provider in this case). Once a Provider becomes aware of such a violation however, the provider has the responsibility of taking reasonable steps to remedy the situation or terminate the contract and inform DHHS as is feasible. The Provider is liable however if the provider does not enter into a Business Associate contract that contains "satisfactory assurances" or if the provider does not take appropriate corrective actions when those assurances are not met.

Many of the provisions of the HIPAA and the HITECH Act apply to Business Associates as well. For example, the privacy and security requirements apply to Business Associates and so do the requirements for notifying violations and breaches. Business Associates are also liable for penalties in case they violate their obligations.

5.4 HIPAA SECURITY RULE

The HIPAA Security Rule pertains to the security of electronic Protected Health Information (ePHI). The focus of the Security Rule is on the integrity and availability of data—i.e., ensuring that it is not modified or lost. The Security Rule is divided into Administrative, Physical and Technical safeguards, which are further divided into standards and specifications. According to this Rule, Covered Entities which "collect, maintain, use or transmit" ePHI must create policies and procedures for "reasonable and appropriate administrative, physical and technical safeguards" to ensure the integrity and availability of data in event of "any reasonably anticipated threats or hazards."

In the following, all quotes are taken directly from the text of HIPAA.

5.4.1 HIPAA Administrative Safeguards

HIPAA Administrative Safeguards are "administrative actions, and policies and procedures, to manage the selection, development, implementation, and maintenance of security measures to protect electronic protected health information (PHI) and to manage the conduct of the Covered Entity's workforce in relation to the protection of that information." They "form the foundation upon which an entity's necessary security activities are built." DHHS requires Covered Entities to take reasonable and appropriate steps to incorporate the Administrative Safeguards while clarifying that "Numerous factors, including ... but not limited to, their size, degree of risk and environment" determine what is reasonable and appropriate. In other words, the specifics of the implementations are left to the judgment of each entity. The implementations however, need to be reviewed and assessed periodically, so that they can be updated in light of emerging risks. This is a continuous process.

The specifications are classified as either "Addressable" or 'Required'. If the specification is 'Required,' the Covered Entity must implement the specification as stated in the Security Rule. If the specification is 'Addressable' the Covered Entity must assess whether the specification is a reasonable and appropriate safeguard in its environment and is likely to contribute to protecting the PHI, document this assessment and if reasonable, implement the specification or an equivalent alternative.

The specifications below need to be implemented by a healthcare provider irrespective of the type of IT solution used (i.e., even by providers who use a Cloud-based solution).

The standards and specifications under Administrative Safeguards are as below.

5.4.1.1 Security Management Process (CFR Section 164.308(a)(1))

Covered entities must implement a security management process as a part of their administrative safeguards. Such a process involves the "implementation of policies and procedures to prevent, detect, contain and correct security violations."

This standard includes four implementation specifications.

5.4.1.1.1 Risk analysis (Required)

Risk Analysis should include "an accurate and thorough assessment of the potential risks and vulnerabilities to the confidentiality, integrity and availability of electronic protected health information (PHI) held by the Covered Entity." Risk Analysis should also estimate the losses that would be incurred due to unauthorized use, disclosure or corruption of PHI.

5.4.1.1.2 Risk management (Required)

Risk management covers the identification and implementation of the security systems and measures which reduce the risks identified above "to a reasonable and appropriate level."

5.4.1.1.3 Sanction policy (Required)

A Sanction policy refers to the disciplinary measures and penalties that would be invoked against the staff members of the healthcare provider should they fail to adhere to the Provider's security procedures and policies. It is up to the provider to determine the quantum and the nature of the penalties for such violations, but they need to be documented a priori.

5.4.1.1.4 Information system activity review (Required)

Information systems activity review is an audit of all logs, incidents and other system activity. The audit should include an implementation of "procedures to regularly review records of information systems activity, such as audit logs, access reports, and security incident tracking reports." The nature and frequency of such audits is not specified, but they need to be conducted regularly, and the results documented. Some of these records and logs are available with the Cloud provider, and need to be obtained from the Cloud-provider in order to perform the necessary review and audits.

5.4.1.2 Assigned Security responsibility (CFR Section 164.308(a) (2)) (Required)

Healthcare providers must designate a "security official," to be "responsible for the development and implementation of the policies and procedures". It is conceivable that in a provider organization, multiple persons handle security responsibilities. Even in such an organization, the designated "security official" must have the final overall responsibility. Even if the provider organization is using a Cloud-based service, it still needs to designate an individual as the Security Officer.

5.4.1.3 Workforce Security (CFR Section 164.308(a)(3))

Healthcare Providers need to ensure the "implementation of policies and procedures to ensure that all members of its workforce have appropriate access to electronic protected health information (PHI)." This translates to access to PHI only on a 'need to know basis'.

The specifications below need to be implemented by the provider even if using a Cloud-based solution.

Workforce security standard has three implementation specifications.

5.4.1.3.1 Authorization and/or supervision (Addressable)

This specification deals with implementation of "procedures for the authorization and/or supervision of workforce members who work with electronic [PHI] or in locations where it might be accessed."

This means that all staff members (physicians, nurse practitioners, administrative personnel, or contract workers) who have access to areas were PHI is stored need to be 'authorized' in order to be there.

5.4.1.3.2 A workforce clearance procedure (Addressable)

Clearance procedures are "procedures to determine that the access of a workforce member to electronic [PHI] is appropriate." Background checks and security vetting is recommended although not mandatory. The Act specifies that "The need for and extent of a screening process is normally based on an assessment of risk, cost, benefit, and feasibility as well as other protective measures in place." Further it is necessary to evaluate the nature of a person's job responsibilities before granting them permission to areas where PHI is stored.

5.4.1.3.3 Termination procedures (Addressable)

This specification refers to "procedures for terminating access to electronic [PHI] when the employment of a workforce member ends" or when the workforce member is reassigned in a manner which no longer requires him/her to access the PHI. This entails steps such as changing access passwords or keys, reprogramming tokens or cards, removal from physical access lists, etc in order to ensure that the workforce member can no longer access the PHI area.

5.4.1.4 Information Access Management (CFR Section 164.308(a) (4))

An information access plan is a set of "policies and procedures for authorizing access to electronic protected health information [PHI]." This involves

5.4.1.4.1 Isolation of any health clearinghouse functions (Required)

HIPAA states that ".... components of a hybrid entity that are designated as health care components must comply with the security standards and protect against unauthorized access with respect to the other components of the larger entity in the same way as they must deal with separate entities."

This is relevant to organizations where PHI related functions relate only to a part of the organization. In this situation the organization needs to put in place barriers to isolate the PHI from persons in the larger organization who are not required to come into contact with PHI.

5.4.1.4.2 Access authorization (Addressable)

This specification pertains to the implementation of policies and procedures that grant access to electronic PHI.

5.4.1.4.3 Access establishment and modification (Addressable)

This specification relates to policies and procedures "that, based upon the entity's access authorization policies, establish, document, review, and modify a user's right of access to a workstation, transaction, program or process."

5.4.1.5 Security Awareness and Training (CFR Section 164.308(a)(5))

Healthcare providers are required to develop a security awareness and training program for their staff including temporary staff "as reasonable and appropriate for them to carry out their functions in the facility." The duration and timing of such training is left to the discretion of the provider. The Act states that the "amount and timing of training should be determined by each Covered Entity; training should be an evolving, on-going process in response to environmental and operational changes". Security awareness and training is necessary even if the practice subscribes to a Cloud-based solution, because several aspects of security pertain to operations performed within the practice.

The following four specifications are defined by this standard:

5.4.1.5.1 Security reminders (Addressable)

Staff members are required to be provided "periodic security updates" and periodically reminded of the security policies and security-related obligations within the organization.

5.4.1.5.2 Protection from malicious software (Addressable)

This includes "procedures for guarding against, detecting and reporting malicious software". This is best ensured by making sure that commercially available anti-malware software (anti-virus, firewalls, etc.) is installed on all computers and upgraded from time to time.

5.4.1.5.3 Log-in monitoring (Addressable)

This includes "procedures for monitoring log-in attempts and reporting discrepancies." If you are using a Cloud-based service, you need to obtain the access logs from your service provider in order to analyze them.

5.4.1.5.4 Password management (Addressable)

This includes "procedures for creating, changing, and safeguarding passwords." Often, Cloud-based services assist in the selection of 'hard' passwords, and prompt users to change passwords from time to time. Providers however need to ensure that the staff members maintain passwords carefully, and not leave them in places where they can be accessed by un-authorized personnel.

5.4.1.6 Security Incident Procedures (CFR Section 164.308(a)(6))

A security incident is "the attempted or successful unauthorized access, use, disclosure, modification, or destruction of information or interference with systems operations in an information system." In spite of safeguards, it is possible that security-related incidents can occur. Healthcare Providers therefore also need to have in place policies and procedures to address security incidents when they do occur. The Cloud-provider needs to inform the practice of any security related incident pertaining to the provider data.

5.4.1.6.1 Response and reporting (Required)

All security incidents need to be handled promptly. This involves the steps of identifying suspected or known security incidents and response thereto, minimizing or eliminating (if possible) the negative impact of the incident, and formal documentation of the incident and its impact.

5.4.1.7 Contingency Plan (CFR Section 164.308(a)(7))

Healthcare providers need to implement a Contingency Plan, i.e., "policies and procedures for responding to an emergency or other occurrence (for example, fire, vandalism, system failure, and natural disaster) that damages systems that contain electronic protected health information [PHI]." The nature of Contingency Plan is provider-specific. The Act states that "Each entity needs to determine its own risk in the event of an emergency that would result in a loss of operations. A contingency plan may involve highly complex processes in one processing site, or simple manual processes in another."

The specifications in this standard include:

5.4.1.7.1 Data backup plan (Required)

This requires Providers "to create and maintain retrievable exact copies of electronic [PHI]." If you are availing of a Cloud-based service, the data backup is typically performed by the Cloud Provider. It is possible for you to request a copy of the data from the provider from time to time or back up the data with another provider.

5.4.1.7.2 Disaster recovery plan (Required)

This requires providers to establish and implement procedures to restore the data from the backup created above. It is necessary to verify that the backup & recovery actually work as expected.

5.4.1.7.3 Emergency mode operation plan (Required)

This requires providers to establish and implement procedures "to enable continuation of critical business processes for protection of the security of ePHI." This means that PHI should remain secured irrespective of natural and man-made emergencies. It is necessary that the provider contractually require the Cloud-vendor to have such an emergency mode operational plan.

5.4.1.7.4 Testing and revision procedures (Addressable)

This specification requires providers to actually test, verify and modify (if required) the emergency and contingency plans put in place for PHI, including plans for backup, recovery and protection of PHI in case of emergencies. How to do this in case of a Cloud-service is discussed in a subsequent chapter.

5.4.1.7.5 Applications and data criticality analysis (Addressable)

This is defined as "assessment of the relative criticality of specific applications and data in support of other contingency plan components."

5.4.1.8 Evaluation (CFR Section 164.308(a)(8)) (Required)

A healthcare provider needs to conduct a "periodic" security evaluation based on the standards specified in the Security Rule, and subsequently on the other "environmental" and "operational" changes that impact the security procedures of the Provider. The "operational" changes are for example changes to IT systems, hiring practices, etc. Providers can either perform such evaluation with an internal resource or hire a consultant to do so.

5.4.1.9 Business Associate Contracts (CFR Section 164.308(b)(1)) (Required)

A healthcare provider can contract with another entity (designated as a Business Associate) to "create, receive, maintain or transmit" PHI for it. The details of who constitutes a Business Associate and the nature of the relationship and contract are already outlined in an earlier section.

This specification requires that Healthcare Providers enter into a Contract with Business Associates. A sample contract is provided in the Appendix. It is also contingent on the healthcare provider, in case of "a pattern of... activity or practice of the business associate that constitute[s] a material breach or violation" do one of the following:

1) Take reasonable steps to halt the breach or end the violation;
2) If such steps are unsuccessful, terminate the contract or arrangement;
3) If termination is not feasible, report the problem to DHHS.

5.4.1.10 Security Policies and Procedures (CFR Section 164.316(a)) (Required)

Healthcare Providers need to implement "reasonable and appropriate policies and procedures to comply with the standards, implementation specifications and other requirements." These are to be "reasonably designed, taking into account the size and type of activities of the Covered Entity that relate to electronic protected health information." These policies and procedures are to be reviewed and updated from time to time, and also documented at all times.

5.4.1.11 Documentation (CFR Section 164.316(b)(1)) (Required)

As mentioned earlier, a Healthcare Provider is required to document all policies, procedures, assessments, activities and actions as specified in the Security Rule. This includes Risk Assessment reports, Action taken reports, designations of responsible persons, Business associate contracts, and so on. All documentation needs to be:

1) Adequately detailed
2) Up-to-date & current at all times after periodic reviews and modifications
3) Always available to those responsible for implementing policies and those who need to know those procedures and policies
4) Preserved for a period of 6 years or the last time it was effective (whichever is longer).

5.4.2 HIPAA Physical safeguards

As per HIPAA Security Rule, physical safeguards are "physical measures, policies and procedures to protect a Covered Entity's electronic information systems and related buildings and equipment, from natural and environmental hazards, and unauthorized intrusion." These are to be implemented by every healthcare provider irrespective of the type of the IT solution employed.

The standards and specifications defined under physical safeguards are as below:

5.4.2.1 Facility Access Controls (CFR Section 164.310(a)(1))

Healthcare providers need to ensure that access to their facilities is controlled and protected. They should incorporate "policies and procedures to limit physical access to its electronic information systems and the facility or facilities in which they are housed, while ensuring that properly authorized access is allowed". Having access control systems fitted on doors with keys/tokens provided to authorized personnel, visitors being recorded and escorted at all times, making note of all goods entering or leaving the premises, are some of the steps that Providers should take.

This covers the following four implementation specifications:

5.4.2.1.1 Contingency operations (Addressable)

This covers "procedures that allow facility access in support of restoration of lost data under the disaster recovery plan and emergency mode operations plan in the event of an emergency."

5.4.2.1.2 Facility security plan (Addressable)

This refers to policies and procedures "to safeguard the facility and the equipment therein from unauthorized physical access, tampering, and theft."

5.4.2.1.3 Access control and validation records (Addressable)

This refers to policies and procedures that "validate a person's [physical] access to facilities based on their role or function, including visitor control, and control of access to software programs for testing and revision." This means that people should have physical access to facilities only on an 'as-required' basis.

5.4.2.1.4 Maintenance records (Addressable)

Providers are required "to document repairs and modifications to the physical components of a facility which are related to security". Such components cover personnel access control systems, including locks, etc.

5.4.2.2 Workstation Use (CFR Section 164.310(b)) (Required)

Providers must incorporate "policies and procedures that specify the proper functions to be performed, the manner in which those functions are to be performed, and the physical attributes of the surroundings of a specific workstation or class of workstation that can access electronic protected health information."

While using Cloud-services, workstations should not be left unattended, and users should 'log off' before leaving the workstation. Here, the term 'workstation' encompasses every device used to access data, including PCs, laptops, hand-held devices, consoles, mobile devices, tablets and so on.

5.4.2.3 Workstation Security (CFR Section 164.310(c)) (Required)

Healthcare Providers need to implement "physical safeguards for all workstations that access electronic protected health information, to restrict access to authorized users."

This means any device that can access PHI either needs to be either in a secure location within the practice or, under the control of authorized personnel at all times.

5.4.2.4 Device and Media Controls (CFR Section 164.310(d)(1))

Healthcare Providers need to implement "policies and procedures that govern the receipt and removal of hardware and electronic media that contain protected health information [PHI] into and out of a facility, and the movement of these items within the facility." This definition covers computers/laptops or handhelds with internal memories that store PHI, as well as storage devices such as internal or external hard disks, USB drives or tapes, etc.

It is possible that you maintain healthcare-related information on storage devices and media even if you subscribe to a Cloud-based solution. The following specifications hence need to be implemented.

Device and Media Controls include four specifications:

5.4.2.4.1 Disposal (Required)

This specification requires implementation of "policies and procedures to address the final disposition of electronic [PHI], and/or the hardware or electronic media on which it is stored."

5.4.2.4.2 Media re-use (Required)

This specification requires policies and procedures for "removal of electronic [PHI] from electronic media before the media are made available for re-use."

5.4.2.4.3 Accountability (Addressable)

This specification requires keeping "a record of the movements of hardware and electronic media and any person responsible therefore."

5.4.2.4.4 Data backup and storage (Addressable)

This specification requires "a retrievable, exact copy of electronic [PHI], when needed, before movement of equipment." This means backing up data before any IT equipment is moved. It is a good idea to periodically backup all data even if you are using a Cloud-based solution.

5.4.3 Technical Safeguards

Technical Safeguards are "the technology and the policy and procedures for its use that protect electronic protected health information [PHI] and control access to it."

The standards and specifications are as below:

5.4.3.1 Access Control (CFR Section 164.312 (a)(1))

This refers to the "technical policies and procedures for electronic information systems access that maintain electronic protected health information [PHI] to allow access only to those persons or software programs that have been granted access rights," i.e., the mechanisms by which access to information is controlled.

The specifications in this standard are as below:

5.4.3.1.1 Unique user identification (Required)

This mandates "assign[ment of] a unique name and/or number for identifying and tracking user identity."

5.4.3.1.2 Emergency access procedure (Required)

This mandates "obtaining necessary [PHI] during an emergency"—a separate specification is necessary because the access to PHI during emergency could be different from access during normal operations.

5.4.3.1.3 Automatic logoff (Addressable)

This mandates mechanisms which "terminate an electronic session after a predetermined time of inactivity." This for example refers to a Cloud-based service logging itself off after a period of inactivity.

5.4.3.1.4 Encryption and decryption (Addressable)

This mandates "mechanism[s] to encrypt and decrypt electronic [PHI]." Encryption/decryption not only refer to data which is stored, but also data which is in transit. This needs to be implemented by the Cloud-solution vendor.

5.4.3.2 Audit Controls (CFR Section 164.312 (b)) (Required)

Healthcare Providers need to ensure "implement[ations] of hardware, software, and/or procedural mechanisms that record and examine activity in information systems that contain or use electronic protected health information [PHI]." However, "Entities have flexibility to implement the standard in a manner appropriate to their needs as deemed necessary by their own risk analyses".

This essentially means an appropriate audit of the activity within the information system that contains PHI. This needs to be implemented by the Cloud-solution vendor.

5.4.3.3 Data Integrity (CFR Section 164.312 (c)(1)) (Addressable)

This standard addresses "policies and procedures to protect electronic protected health information [PHI] from improper alteration or destruction." The implementation specification requires providers to "[I]mplement electronic mechanisms to corroborate that electronic [PHI] has not been altered or destroyed in an unauthorized manner."

The most common technologies to ensure data integrity are based on cryptographic hash algorithms, and commercially available products need to be utilized to ensure that PHI is not altered either when stored or in transit. This needs to be implemented by the Cloud-solution vendor.

5.4.3.4 Person or Entity authentication (CFR Section 164.312 (d)) (Required)

Providers are required to ensure "implement[ation] of procedures to verify that a person or entity seeking access to electronic protected health information [PHI] is the one claimed." There are several technologies that ensure identity verification, and any of these may be deployed to verify the identity of an individual before sharing PHI.

5.4.3.5 Transmission and Security (CFR Section 164.312 (e)(1))

Providers also need to ensure the security of data in transit, defined as "technical security mechanisms to guard against unauthorized access to electronic protected health information [PHI] that is being transmitted over an electronic communications network." The transmitted information could refer to information being communicated to a Business Associate, to the patient or any other situation requiring transmission of PHI.

The following two specifications are defined, both of which need to be implemented by the Cloud vendor:

5.4.3.5.1 Integrity controls (Addressable)

This covers "security measures to ensure that electronically transmitted electronic protected health information is not improperly modified without detection until disposed of." Essentially meaning that it is necessary to ensure that the information in transit is not modified.

5.4.3.5.2 Encryption (Addressable)

This requires implementation of "mechanisms to encrypt electronic [PHI] deemed appropriate." While the specific technologies are not specified, it is advisable to encrypt all data (stored or in transit) with commercial grade encryption and use cryptographic hash algorithms.

5.5 HIPAA PRIVACY RULE

The HIPAA Privacy rule lays down standards and guidelines for the protecting the privacy of healthcare information.

On one hand, any unauthorized disclosure of healthcare information is a violation of individuals' privacy rights. On the other hand we have seen how transfer of health information can actually promote better health care and patient's well being. In certain circumstances, sharing healthcare information may also be required to protect public health.

It is therefore necessary to strike a balance—i.e., lay down guidelines on how personal health information is to be protected, and at the same time define the circumstances under which it can be shared or transferred along with the method in which this may be done.

The Privacy rule provides this balance. Not only does it specify how an individual's PHI is to be protected, but also defines the circumstances in which it may be disclosed and shared by Covered Entities.

5.5.1 Who is covered by the Privacy Rule

Privacy Rule protections extend to every patient whose information is collected, used or disclosed by Covered Entities. The obligations of the Privacy Rule apply to all Covered Entities that come into contact with healthcare information. This includes:

1) Health Plans that pay or provide for the cost of medical services. This includes for example, health plans, dental plans, vision and prescription drug insurers, health maintenance organizations (HMO), Medicare, Medicaid, long-term care insurers, employer-sponsored group health plans, multi-employer health plans, etc. It also applies to their employees, volunteers and consultants.

2) Healthcare Providers which includes every entity that provides healthcare related services. It includes institutional providers such as hospitals, clinics, etc of any size, including their employees, volunteers and their consultants. It also applies to individual providers such as physicians, dentists, nurses and other healthcare practitioners.

3) Healthcare Clearinghouses that process healthcare information, and includes entities such as billing service companies, repricing companies, community health management information systems, and other healthcare information networks.

4) Business Associates are also covered by the Privacy Rule. We have noted that Covered Entities need to enter into contracts with Business Associates which include assurances & provisions for the protection of Healthcare information in the same manner that the Covered Entity itself protects such information.

5.5.2 What kind of information is protected?

Under the Privacy Rule, Protected Health Information refers to all "individually identifiable health information held or transmitted by a Covered Entity or its business associate, in any form or media, whether electronic, paper, or oral."

"Individually identifiable health information" is information, including demographic data, that relates to:

1) The individual's past, present or future physical or mental health or condition,
2) The provision of health care to the individual, or
3) The past, present, or future payment for the provision of health care to the individual, and that identifies the individual or for which there is a reasonable basis to believe can be used to identify the individual.

Information that contains for example the name, address, birth date, Social Security Number, etc. of the patient is called "Individually identifiable health information"

The Provisions do not apply to "De-identified Health Information", which means information that does not identify the patient or provide a basis to identify the patient. Information can be de-identified by removing all identifying information such as the name, address, date of birth, social security number, information about relatives, employer, etc.

5.5.3 Individual Rights

The Privacy Rule assigns several rights to the patient including:

1) Patients are required to be given a Notice of its Privacy Practices by the Covered Entity. This notice needs to provide information about the Privacy Practices followed by the Covered Entity and how the Covered Entity shall use and disclose protected health information.
2) Patients have the right to access and obtain copies of their own health records.
3) Patients have the right to request correction or amendment to their healthcare information if they find it to be erroneous or incomplete.

4) Patients have the right to obtain an accounting of all disclosures in the past 6 years, i.e., list of entities including individuals and organizations to whom their personal health information has been disclosed in the past 6 years. This however, does not cover certain types of disclosures, including those related to providing treatment, disclosures made to law enforcement, disclosures made to the patient or their representatives, and other disclosures as allowed by the rule.

5) Patients can request restrictions on certain information - for example restrictions on access, use or disclosure of specific information, although the Covered Entity is under no obligation to agree to such a restriction if it informs the Patient accordingly.

6) Patients can request that communication regarding their health information be made by alternative means or at alternative locations. Providers are required to accommodate reasonable requests if the patient indicates that the disclosure of health information could endanger the patient.

7) Covered Entities need to designate a Privacy Officer and share the name and contact information of the Privacy Officer in the Notice of Privacy Practices provided to Patients. Patients can complain to the Privacy Officer in case of any problems. Patients can further pursue the complaint with the US Department of Health and Human Services' Office of Civil Rights if the problems are not satisfactorily resolved.

5.5.4 Permitted Uses and Disclosures

There are several situations under which PHI may need to be disclosed. Following are some examples of situations where disclosure is permitted:

1) A Covered Entity is required to disclose PHI to the patient (or their representatives) and to HHS when requested.

2) A Covered Entity is permitted to use and disclose protected health information, after providing the initial Privacy Notice, for the purpose of treatment, payment, and healthcare operations. Treatment refers to provision and management of healthcare and related services by one or more health care providers, including consultation between providers or patient

referral. Payment refers to activities of the Covered Entity to obtain payment or be reimbursed for the provision of health care to the patient. Healthcare Operations encompasses a variety of operations such as quality assessment, competency evaluation, medical reviews, audits, general administrative activities, etc.

3) A Covered Entity may obtain informal permission by asking the individual, or by giving the individual the opportunity to agree, acquiesce, or object to sharing certain information. In emergency situations or circumstances where the individual is incapacitated, the attending physician or nurse may make a professional judgment about disclosure of information that would be in the best interest of the patient. The information that may be shared after such informal permission includes information required for facilities listing and for notification purposes.

4) A Covered Entity may obtain separate authorization from the patient for sharing information for the purposes of research, marketing or fundraising.

5) A Covered Entity may disclose PHI without patient authorization for the purposes of public health & safety, law enforcement, health oversight, judicial or administrative proceedings, and if required by law for any reason.

5.5.5 Administrative requirements

There are several administrative requirements imposed upon a Covered Entity by the HIPAA Privacy rule. All of these apply even when using a Cloud-based IT solution. These include:

1) *Privacy Policies and Procedures.* A Covered Entity must develop and implement written privacy policies and procedures consistent with the Privacy Rule.

2) *Privacy Personnel.* Each Covered Entity must designate a 'privacy official' who shall be responsible for developing and implementing its privacy policies and procedures. There will also need to be designated a contact official for receiving complaints and providing individuals with information on the Covered Entity's privacy practices.

3) *Workforce Training and Management.* Workforce members include employees, volunteers, trainees, and may also include other persons whose conduct is under the direct control of the Covered Entity. A Covered Entity must train all workforce members on its privacy policies and procedures, as necessary and appropriate for them to carry out their functions. A Covered Entity must have and apply appropriate sanctions against workforce members who violate its privacy policies and procedures or the Privacy Rule.

4) *Mitigation.* A Covered Entity must mitigate, to the extent possible, any harmful effect it learns were caused by use or disclosure of protected health information by its workforce or its business associates in violation of its privacy policies and procedures or the Privacy Rule.

5) *Data Safeguards.* A Covered Entity must maintain reasonable and appropriate administrative, technical, and physical safeguards to prevent intentional or unintentional use or disclosure of protected health information in violation of the Privacy Rule and to limit its incidental use and disclosure pursuant to otherwise permitted or required use or disclosure. For example, such safeguards might include shredding documents containing protected health information before discarding them, securing medical records with lock and key or pass code, and limiting access to those keys or pass codes.

6) *Complaints.* A Covered Entity must have procedures for individuals to complain about its compliance with its privacy policies and procedures and the Privacy Rule. The Covered Entity must explain those procedures in its privacy practices notice.

7) *Retaliation and Waiver.* A Covered Entity may not retaliate against a person for exercising rights provided by the Privacy Rule, for assisting in an investigation by DHHS or other appropriate authority, or for opposing an act or practice that the person believes violates the Privacy Rule. A Covered Entity may not require an individual to waive any right under the Privacy Rule as a condition for obtaining treatment, payment, and enrollment or benefits eligibility.

8) *Documentation and Record Retention.* A Covered Entity must maintain, until six years after the later of the date of their creation or last effective date, its privacy policies and procedures, its privacy practices notices, disposition of complaints, and other actions, activities, and designations that the Privacy Rule requires to be documented.

5.6 HIPAA BEST PRACTICES

The Office of E-Health Standards & Services (which is a part of CMS) conducted audit of several organizations in 2008 for compliance with the Security Rule. It published a report titled "HIPAA Compliance Review Analysis and Summary of Results," which outlined its findings [9].

The report suggests that provider organizations are often found lacking in aspects such as conducting background checks on employees before they are given access to PHI, training of personnel on security compliance issues, ensuring the security of computers, ensuring that all information policies and procedures are up-to-date and complied with, and ensuring that all data within the provider organization (whether it is stored or in transit) is properly encrypted.

5.6.1 Risk assessment

Healthcare Providers are required to undertake a risk assessment of their operations from time to time, create a 'Risk Assessment Document', and then take actions in order to eliminate perceived risks to the privacy and security of healthcare data. If you are using a Cloud-based Service, virtually all of your data storage and processing happens outside of your premises, on systems that are controlled by the Cloud Provider. However, you are still required to conduct a risk assessment to ensure the compliance of your organization with HIPAA. It is therefore necessary to know what such an assessment entails and how it benefits your organization.

Healthcare organizations are required to "Conduct accurate and thorough assessment of the potential risks and vulnerabilities to the confidentiality, integrity, and availability of electronic protected health information (ePHI) held by the Covered Entity." This is known as a Risk Assessment.

CMS Recommends the following solution [9]:

1) Covered Entities (CE) should develop and formally document a policy requiring the completion of a periodic risk assessment covering all systems and applications which store, process, or transmit ePHI (electronic PHI). Risk assessments should be completed every three years or sooner if there is a significant change in the environment such as introduction or upgrades to existing systems, relocation, disposal of systems, or change in business including commencement of new lines of business.

2) CEs should identify the systems which store, process, or transmit ePHI, identify components of the organization (human resources) which handle ePHI, their physical location and location of IT assets. Thereafter, the CE should.

   i. Identify the criticality of the system and its data;

   ii. Identify threats to the system;

   iii. Identify vulnerabilities on the system;

   iv. Analyze the controls that have been implemented, or are planned for implementation;

   v. Identify the probability that vulnerability may be exploited;

   vi. Identify the impact of a successful threat exercise;

   vii. Assess the level of risk;

   viii. Identify additional controls to mitigate identified risks; and,

   ix. Document the results of the risk assessment.

3) CEs should conduct a formal, documented Risk Assessment for systems and applications which store, process, or transmit ePHI. This can be done using a 'Risk Assessment Matrix'. The resulting Risk Assessment should be approved by management. The approver should not be the individual responsible for completing the risk assessment or involved with the day to day operation of the assessed system. CEs should retain evidence of this approval, within the document itself if possible.

After CEs complete their Risk Assessment, they should identify corrective actions for any weaknesses they identify during the process. They should also identify steps to mitigate the residual risks identified in the risk assessment. If risks are scored by their probabilities and 'impact scores' (estimated impact of the vulnerability on the organization), it is best to begin by addressing the risks that have the highest probability of occurrence or a high 'impact-score'. The CE needs to create a plan for implementation of corrective measures including physical and technical safeguards to protect PHI.

4) Each CE needs to designate an individual as the Chief Compliance Officer who shall be responsible for ensuring compliance of the organization with the Security and Privacy rule provisions of HIPAA. It is the duty of this person to sign off on the Risk Assessment document, identify corrective actions and ensure their implementation. This person will also be responsible for responding to the CMS in case of an audit. This person may not conduct the Risk Assessment himself/herself, but the person assumes overall responsibility for compliance.

There are many resources available that can help your practice conduct a Risk Assessment. For example, the American Health Care Association provides several resources which detail how a Risk Assessment is to be performed [10]. Similarly the American Health Information Management Association [11] has resources for conducting a Risk Assessment for your practice. However, conducting a Risk Assessment usually requires a team of experts with technical knowledge of the functioning of the IT systems, including knowledge of software and hardware. If this knowledge is not present internally within the practice (as is most likely the case), the Risk Assessment is best done by an external expert.

There are several consulting firms that can conduct a Risk Assessment for your practice. These consulting firms not only create a Risk Assessment report, but also work with you to implement remedial measures when vulnerability is detected. Outsourcing the task to a consultant can be a viable option especially because such consultants normally have experience of conducting similar assessments at various other practices. Further, they can bring a fresh perspective to the policies and procedures of your practice.

5.6.2 Currency of Policies and Procedures

It is necessary that CE policies and procedures be upgraded from time to time, and the upgrades documented. HIPAA requires Covered Entities to "Perform a periodic technical and nontechnical evaluation, based initially upon the standards implemented under this rule, and subsequently, in response to environmental or operational changes affecting the security of electronic protected health information that establishes the extent to which an entity's security policies and procedures meet the requirements of this subpart." The Security Rule emphasizes the importance of "continued effectiveness of security processes driven by documented policies and procedures". Although the frequency of such evaluation is not specified, it is clear that the creation of policies and their compliance should be an on-going activity.

Specifically, Covered Entities need to:

1) Review and approve security policies and procedures within appropriate time frame
2) Document evidence of their review and approval of policies and procedures
3) Document procedures that are consistent with procedures followed by personnel.

The CMS report recommends that:

1) CEs should develop and formally document a policy requiring that management periodically review policies and procedures. This policy should outline the maximum timeframe between reviews as well as require management review when there is a significant change to systems or the environment.
2) CEs should develop and formally document a procedure for conducting periodic reviews of policies and procedures. This procedure should allow management to conduct these reviews in a timely manner, compliant with the CE's documented policy for frequency of this type of review. The process should outline the steps for management to:
   i. Identify policies and procedures for which they are responsible for reviewing;

    ii. Gather the most recent versions of these policies and procedures;

    iii. Assess the currency of the documented policy or procedure against the organization's operational and regulatory environment;

    iv. Implement updates to the policy or procedure as necessary;

    v. Document evidence of their review and approval; and,

    vi. Disseminate the updated policy or procedure throughout the organization.

3) CEs should develop a standard format for documenting policies and procedures. This format should accommodate multiple types of documents, but should maintain information on revisions to the document, the dates of each revision, the individual who revised the document, the date of the most recent approval of the document, and the individual who approved it.

4) CEs should evaluate their process for disseminating and adopting updated policies and procedures to determine if employees are aware of updates. As part of this process, CEs should develop tools to manage policies and procedures as well as aid management with their review. Ideally, these tools should allow individuals to register for automated notifications when management updates policies or procedures. In addition, updates to organization-wide policies and procedures should be communicated to all employees. These updates should be reiterated in refresher security awareness training.

5) CEs should conduct periodic evaluations, either internally or by engaging a third party, to assess the effectiveness of policies and procedures and their compliance with the Security Rule. CEs can perform this assessment through a number of methods including interviews, process walkthroughs, and/or assessment of the actual results of these processes. Larger organizations should consider a formalized review conducted by internal audit. Smaller organizations should consider less formal means of evaluation or engagement of a third party. The individuals who conduct these evaluations should not be the same as those

responsible for carrying out the process and should maintain a reasonable level of competence to properly perform the assessment.

5.6.3 Workforce Clearance, Security Awareness and Training

Covered Entities are required to "Implement procedures to determine that the access of a workforce member to electronic protected health information is appropriate." CEs need to complete background investigation check on their employees prior to providing them access to ePHI. CEs should also require background investigations from vendors and third parties who have access to ePHI. This should be part of the requirements established in Business Associate Agreements with these vendors and third parties. Access should be restricted to only those individuals who have a reasonable need to utilize the ePHI.

It is necessary that the staff (including physicians, nurse practitioners, administrative personnel and anyone else with access to PHI) within a Healthcare provider organization be trained on HIPAA, particularly its Privacy and Security rules. This is required even if the Provider is using a Cloud-based solution. Such training is not only administered as a part of the employee's orientation process, i.e., before the employee commences work, but also periodically from time to time whenever there is a change in regulations.

There are numerous third-party consultants that conduct HIPAA training for your staff. Details of these consultants can be located by searching on the Internet. Many of these training modules are available online, and can be availed by staff members at their convenience.

Typical HIPAA training covers modules such as:

1) Overview of HIPAA
2) Administrative requirements
3) The reasons for HIPAA Security & Privacy Rules
4) HIPAA Security & Privacy Rules
5) The responsibilities & obligations of healthcare staff under HIPAA

6) Precautions & Safeguards while working with Healthcare information
7) Conditions under which Healthcare Information can be disclosed
8) Patient rights
9) Liabilities and Penalties
10) Best practices to guard against inadvertent disclosure of healthcare data
11) Examples of real-life scenarios

The above training is necessary even when you are using a Cloud-based service. Further, it is necessary that the you designate a Chief Compliance Officer who may be approached by staff in case of doubts.

5.6.4 Workstation Security and Encryption

HIPAA requires that CEs "Implement physical safeguards for all workstations that access electronic protected health information, to restrict access to authorized users." These standards stress the importance of protecting workstations that store, process, or transmit ePHI.

In order to enhance compliance with the Security Rule, the following solutions are recommended [9]:

1) CEs should develop a policy outlining workstation classifications and the types of physical security controls the CE requires for each class of workstations. This policy should take into consideration the results of the Risk Assessment to identify threat sources and potential environments where workstations exist.
2) CEs should develop a policy for performing security walkthrough. This policy should identify a specific timeframe for performing the reviews, the types of reviews the CE will perform, and the scope of the walkthroughs (e.g. facility locations or specific areas of single facilities). CEs should consider identifying sensitive areas in their facilities which require additional scrutiny.

3) CEs should develop procedures for the types of walkthroughs they perform in their environment. These procedures should specify the steps for performing walkthroughs as well as documenting the results of each walkthrough. This documentation should include details regarding who performed the walkthrough, the date the individual performed the walkthrough, and the results of the process.

4) CEs should evaluate the results of the walkthroughs. The results can then be used to identify areas where the CE may need to deploy additional employee training or physical security controls.

5) CEs should outline physical security requirements in initial and refresher security awareness training. The training should specifically outline employees' responsibility for securing workstations, laptops, and other portable devices.

Further, HIPAA requires that CEs "Implement a mechanism to encrypt and decrypt electronic protected health information", and further that "all portable or remote devices that store ePHI employ encryption technologies of the appropriate strength... Deploy policy to encrypt backup and archival media; ensure that policies direct the use of encryption technologies of the appropriate strength."

In order to increase compliance with this element of the Security Rule, the following solutions are recommended [9]: [Note: If you are using a Cloud-based vendor encrypting the data is the responsibility of the vendor, however, if you keep a copy of data with you, the guidelines pertaining to encryption need to be followed].

1) CEs should develop an accurate inventory of laptops, workstations, and other portable devices or media. Failure to establish an accurate inventory usually results in the lack of assurance that CEs have encrypted all devices which require this protection. Maintenance of this inventory should be integrated with the procurement process for new systems and devices.

2) CEs should develop and formally document policies requiring encryption of ePHI. The policy should address situations where encryption is required. These situations should be identified based on risk. In addition, the policy should outline the minimum level of encryption required for ePHI at rest and in transit.

3) CEs should implement an encryption solution on all workstations and laptops which store, process, or transmit ePHI. Because of the ease with which electronic data moves between systems, CEs should also consider extending these protections to all workstations and laptops. The software should provide a whole disk encryption solution using strong encryption technology. If possible, the solution should be validated as compliant with Federal Information Processing Standards (FIPS) Publication (Pub) 140-2, "Security Requirements for Cryptographic Modules" or leverage encryption modules which validate as compliance.

4) CEs should identify requirements for encryption of portable devices and media as necessary. If ePHI is stored on USB keys, backup tapes, PDA, Blackberries, iPods, or other portable devices, the data on this media should be encrypted. CEs should also consider implementing policies specifically forbidding ePHI on these types of devices; however, CEs must then consider approaches to prevent this information from moving to these devices. Such a decision will be dependent on the work of the employees, and the need to be able to access data from a portable device, particularly in the clinical arena, given the advent of electronic health records and personal health records which are designed to be accessed from anywhere at any time.

5) CEs should implement strong encryption on wireless networks, if they are used to transmit ePHI. Wireless networking technology continues to evolve, as does the security around these networks. Because of longstanding identified weaknesses in WEP and recently identified in WPA using TKIP8, organizations must research encryption methods which reasonably and appropriately protect ePHI in transit. These mechanisms should be revisited as wireless security evolves.

6) CEs should communicate encryption requirements to the workforce through policies, initial security awareness training, and periodic refresher training. Training should include information on employee responsibilities as they relate to encryption, and should be updated based on new threats to encrypted data. Changes in the threat environment introduce additional risk which CEs must identify and mitigate.

7) After CEs implement encryption, they should update their system baselines and build procedures to reflect the deployment of the encryption solutions.

5.7 BREACH NOTIFICATION

The HITECH Act holds healthcare providers (and their business associates) accountable for ensuring the privacy and security of healthcare data entrusted to their care. A 'breach' is said to have occurred when an individual's Protected Health Information is disclosed by a provider (or a Business Associate) to entities to which it was not to be disclosed. To quote the Act, a breach "[is an] unauthorized acquisition, access, use or disclosure of PHI which compromises the security or privacy of the PHI, except where an unauthorized person to whom such information is disclosed would not reasonably have been able to retain such information."

When such a breach is discovered the Provider is required to notify the individual whose Health information has been disclosed. In addition, the Provider is also required to inform the FTC (Federal Trade Commission). If a Business Associate is responsible for the disclosure, the Business Associate is in addition required to notify the Provider of the breach. Such a notification should include:

1) A description of the breach incident, including its date and also the date of discovery.
2) A description of the type of health information that was disclosed (such as any information that can be used to identify the patient, information about the nature of the illness, diagnosis, or other such clinical or non-clinical information).
3) Suggested steps the individual can take to protect themselves from harmful effects resulting from the breach.
4) A description of the steps the provider/Business Associate is taking to investigate the breach, minimize its impact and guard against the possibility of future breaches.
5) Contact information and procedure whereby the affected individual can obtain further information about the breach, including a toll-free phone number, email address, web-site or postal address.

Breach Notification obligations do not apply in the following situations (Exceptions to the breach Notification Rule):

1) If the health Information is 'secured', i.e., encrypted as per standards laid down, its disclosure is exempted from the requirement of notification

2) If the entity to which the information is disclosed is unable to store or retain the disclosed information, its disclosure is exempted from notification

3) If the individual to whom disclosure happens is an employee or acting under the authority of the Covered Entity or business associate.

4) If the individual to whom disclosure is made is authorized to handle protected health information (for example during a referral to another physician).

Breach Notifications have to be made within 60 days of the discovery of the breach either by first class mail or by email if specified by the individual. If 500 or more individuals are impacted, the DHHS should be notified immediately. If more than 500 individuals of a single jurisdiction are impacted, a press release regarding the breach needs to be issued via media outlets.

The rules and regulations pertaining to breach Notification can change from time to time, and the latest information is can be accessed from the HHS website [12].

5.8 EHR REGIONAL EXTENSION CENTERS

The HITECH Act recognizes the challenges that healthcare providers are likely to face in the selection and adoption of EHR systems. For this reason, the HITECH Act envisages the setting up of "Health Information Technology Regional Extension Centers" and also sets aside financial assistance for them. As per the Act, the purpose of these regional centers is "to provide technical assistance and disseminate best practices and other information to support and accelerate efforts to adopt, implement, and effectively utilize health information technology that allows for the electronic exchange and use of information in compliance with standards, implementation specifications, and certification criteria..." The Act further states that

"The objective of the regional centers is to enhance and promote the adoption of health information technology through—

"(A) assistance with the implementation, effective use, upgrading, and ongoing maintenance of health information technology, including electronic health records, to healthcare providers nationwide;

"(B) broad participation of individuals from industry, universities, and State governments;

"(C) active dissemination of best practices and research on the implementation, effective use, upgrading, and ongoing maintenance of health information technology, including electronic health records, to health care providers in order to improve the quality of healthcare and protect the privacy and security of health information;

"(D) participation, to the extent practicable, in health information exchanges;

"(E) utilization, when appropriate, of the expertise and capability that exists in Federal agencies other than the Department; and

"(F) integration of health information technology, including electronic health records, into the initial and ongoing training of health professionals and others in the healthcare industry that would be instrumental to improving the quality of healthcare through the smooth and accurate electronic use and exchange of health information."

These regional centers are expected to provide assistance to healthcare providers in a specific geographical region, and can be approached by any healthcare provider within that region for assistance.

5.9 ENFORCEMENT

Although HIPAA has existed for several years, its provisions have not always been strictly enforced. The HITECH Act suggests that it will be rigorously enforced. The Act contains penalties for "willful neglect", which can run into hundreds of thousands of dollars with penalties for repeat violations going up to $1.5 million. It is therefore necessary that providers are able to demonstrate a genuine effort to comply with the provisions of law. It is to be noted that the HHS is now required to conduct audits at regular intervals of healthcare providers, with providers being required to demonstrate compliance.

5.10 MEANINGFUL USE CRITERIA

The DHHS released on July 13 2010 the final rule establishing the criteria for meaningful use of electronic health records under the Medicare and Medicaid incentive programs [13]. The DHHS also simultaneously released the final rule to establish initial data standards, implementation specifications and certification criteria for electronic health records. These final rules are included as appendices to the book.

The rule for "meaningful use" specifies 15 base requirements which healthcare providers have to meet. Additionally they have to meet 5 more requirements out of 10 additional options provided. Aiming to lower the hurdles, the finalized rules require that providers meet 14 to 15 base requirements and choose five more from a menu of 10 options. The core objectives of these criteria are the "basic functions that enable EHRs to support improved healthcare" [14]. To further quote from [14].

"As a start, these include the tasks essential to creating any medical record, including the entry of basic data: Patients' vital signs and demographics, active medications and allergies, up-to-date problem lists of current and active diagnoses and smoking status,"

"Other core objectives include using several software applications that begin to realize the true potential of EHRs to improve the safety, quality, and efficiency of care. These features help clinicians to make better clinical decisions and avoid preventable errors."

The menu of 10 additional tasks includes "capacities to perform drug-formulary checks, incorporate clinical laboratory results into EHRs, provide reminders to patients for needed care, identify and provide patient-specific health education resources, and employ

EHRs to support the patient's transitions between care settings or personnel," the pair wrote.

None of the 15 base requirements are such that they cannot be met by Cloud-based solutions. Additionally, Cloud-based solutions will be in a position to support optional requirements as well.

Practitioners who opt for Cloud-based solutions should ensure however that the solutions are certified as per the certification criteria provided by DHHS in [13].

REFERENCES

[1] US Government Printing Office Website (http://frwebgate.access.gpo.gov/cgi-bin/getdoc.cgi?dbname=104_cong_public_laws&docid=f:publ191.104)

[2] http://www.legalarchiver.org/hipaa.htm

[3] http://www.hhs.gov/ocr/privacy/

[4] https://www.cms.gov/hipaageninfo/

[5] Redhead, C.S. Medical records privacy: Questions and answers on the HIPAA final rule (CRS Report for Congress, Order Code RS20500). Washington, DC: Congressional Research Service, Library of Congress, 2001.

[6] Subtitle A, Public Law 111-5

[7] http://www.hhs.gov/ocr/privacy/hipaa/understanding/coveredentities/contractprov.html

[8] http://www.medlawplus.com/forminfo/hipaaprivacyagreement.htm

[9] http://www.hhs.gov/ocr/privacy/hipaa/enforcement/cmscompliancerev08.pdf

[10] http://www.ahcancal.org/facility_operations/hipaa/Pages/HIPAARiskAssessmentSecurityTools.aspx

[11] http://www.ahima.org

[12] http://www.hhs.gov

[13] http://www.ofr.gov/OFRUpload/OFRData/2010-17210_PI.pdf

[14] The *Meaningful Use* Regulation for Electronic Health Records, by David Blumenthal and Marilyn Tavenner, New England Journal of Medicine, 2010.

CHAPTER 6

Adopting Cloud Services

In this chapter, we will discuss the stages involved in the successful selection and adoption of a Cloud-based IT solution. The following, broadly are the stages in the process:

1) The first stage involves ascertaining definitively that a Cloud-based offering is indeed the most suitable for your practice from among the number of options available. Procuring and implementing an IT solution is not only time consuming but also involves significant involvement of organization's personnel. Furthermore, although it is possible, it is certainly not easy to change your IT solution once a particular solution has been installed. Functionality and ease of use are two of the most important factors that impact practitioner's choice of IT systems and evaluating these requires actually trying out the products. There are a few hundred healthcare IT solutions available in the market today with in-house software and Cloud-based solutions being the two primary categories of solutions. It is a good idea to make the cloud vs. non-cloud decision first and then evaluate products within that category. If a suitable solution can't be located in the preferred category, the practitioner can then look at the other category. Therefore, identifying whether you want to go the cloud route is a good first step.

2) If, and once you decide to opt for a Cloud-based solution, it is necessary to install and test the basic infrastructure that you will need to utilize a Cloud service. While the required infrastructure is significantly less than what is required for an

in-house solution, the computers and the network required to access the Cloud service need to be put in place. Prior installation and use of that infrastructure for non-critical Cloud-based applications is useful to ensure that there are no setbacks when the same infrastructure is subsequently used for a mission-critical Cloud-based healthcare IT system.

3) The third stage involves identification and selection of a Cloud-based solution vendor that best meets the requirements of your practice. This stage can be undertaken in parallel with the installation and testing of your internal IT setup (stage 2). Needless to say, there are numerous vendors who offer Cloud-based solutions which you will consider as potential candidates for your organization. Not only should you identify as many vendor options as possible, but also have a process and checklists in place for determining which of the vendor's solution is most appropriate for you.

4) Finally, once a vendor is selected, you need to create a 'transition road-map' for your organization. This means moving to the Cloud-based offering from your existing solution. With on-site systems, the solution vendors normally provide on-site consulting to help you manage the transition to their software. With Cloud-based offerings, such on-site consulting may or may not be available—either you will need to work with independent consultants to manage the transition or allocate resources within your practice to do so.

The following are some of the common observations based on the experience of practices that have conducted any type of migration of IT systems (whether it is from paper to EMR, or in-house to Cloud-based or a change of provider).

1) As in any discipline, there is usually a resistance to change existing systems or procedures. There is skepticism about potential benefits of making any change. The fact that there are financial incentives for adoption of EMR will probably minimize some of this skepticism, but it is absolutely essential to obtain a buy-in from all stake-holders (all potential users) before any migration is planned. Arriving at such a consensus usually involves multiple meetings among stakeholders and can take time.

2) In smaller practices, it is vital to have *all* physicians and nurse practitioners agree on the need to make the transition, and it is best if key decisions on migration (vendor selection, actual migration process, etc) are made by physicians. In other words probability of success is maximized if the physicians are the primary drivers of the transition.

3) Practices which involve more than 10 users find it convenient to form a smaller team of 'super-users' which basically is a team of representatives which includes physicians, nurse practitioners, administrative staff etc. who will evaluate systems, make a selection, manage the migration process, function as in-house consultants on system use and in general champion the transition to the Cloud-based system. This ensures that not everyone needs to be involved with the time-consuming process of system evaluation and selection.

6.1 CLOUD-BASED SOLUTIONS VS. IN-HOUSE SYSTEMS

The pros and cons of Cloud-based solutions have been considered in detail in chapter 2. The key concerns about Cloud-based services pertain to their availability and security. Their primary advantages pertain to costs, and ease of use. The perception and relative importance of these pros and cons are likely to differ for each user. Similarly, each user group/practice is likely to have a different level of inherent comfort with using a cloud offering.

A Cloud-based solution should definitely be considered by smaller clinics and practices if they can identify one that meets the functional requirements of their specialty.

6.2 GETTING STARTED WITH A NON-CRITICAL CLOUD-BASED SERVICE (CREATING THE INFRASTRUCTURE)

A large part of using a Cloud-based healthcare IT solution has to do with the comfort level with using *any* Cloud-based service at all. If you have only recently been introduced to the concept of a Cloud it is not easy to accept the idea of all your data being stored at a location outside your premises. It is also important to determine if it is possible to setup the type of internet infrastructure in your clinic that is required to use a Cloud-based service.

It is a good idea for decision-makers/IT users within the practice to answer the following questions before they decide to sign up with a Cloud-based service.

1) Do you use any web based services such as web-email or social networking sites?
2) Do you conduct bank financial transactions over the Internet?
3) Do you have Internet connectivity in your office? Are you able to connect to the Internet from your office virtually anytime you want to?
4) Do you know other practices that have been using Cloud-based healthcare IT solutions?

If you have *not* answered a YES to at least 3 of the above 4 questions, the first step should be to commence using a Cloud-based service for your corporate email (Several vendors, for example Google, have Cloud-based email) solutions that your practice can subscribe to). If you do not have an internet connection to your office, you should identify and sign up with an internet provider for an internet connection.

Before signing up with a Cloud-based healthcare IT solution, you should put the infrastructure in place and use it to access non-critical web-services for at least 3 months.

This involves the following:

6.2.1 Selecting and signing up with Internet Service provider(s)

Here is a list of questions to ask a prospective internet vendor before making a selection:

1) What is the type of technology (wired/wireless/cable)? If it is a wired connection, will a connection be available immediately? If it's a wireless technology, what is the quality of received signal at your particular location? What is the sort of equipment that will be housed on your premises? It is true that the technology used by your Internet provider does not really matter while actually using the Cloud service. The reason for asking these questions however is to verify that it does not require installation of too many pieces of equipment on your premises, and secondly to ensure that the two

internet connections you eventually subscribe to are based on two different technologies. So, for example, if one of your two connections is a optic fiber line, it is a good idea for your second connection to be a wireless link.

2) What is the upload speed and the download speed of the connection? Note that for most Internet connections, the download speed is 4–6 times the upload speed. While using an Internet connection for healthcare IT, it is best to have a good download speed (at least 5 mbps for a small practice) and at least a moderate upload speed (at least 1Mbps).

3) Average availability statistics (if any). Are their statistics available for the uptime/downtime of the Internet service?

4) Are there other businesses in the neighborhood who have obtained an Internet connection from the same provider, and if so, what is their experience?

5) What are the monthly connection plans (Unlimited usage, metered, etc)? It is usually good to sign up with an unlimited usage plan if one is not sure of the anticipated level of one's usage.

6) Does the provider provide a connection with a Static IP address or a dynamic IP? Having a static IP address is useful for the purpose of auditing user logs of a Cloud service and also for controlling access (if facility exists) to your Cloud account.

7) What is the latency of your connection? The latency, which refers to any type of delays associated with your data travelling on the network impacts the speed of loading a standard web-page in your browser. Latency can be determined using ping tests. A latency of less than 100 milliseconds is preferred.

It is best to procure two (fully redundant) internet connections for your practice, i.e., two connections from two vendors based on two different technologies. It is best to have your IT consultant configure them for automatic switchover. This means that both the external connections are terminated into a single switch, and the computers within your facility can access the internet on either of the two connections. When one of the internet services fails, all internet traffic is automatically routed over the other service without any configuration or setup changes on part of the users. The configuration is shown in Fig. 6.1.

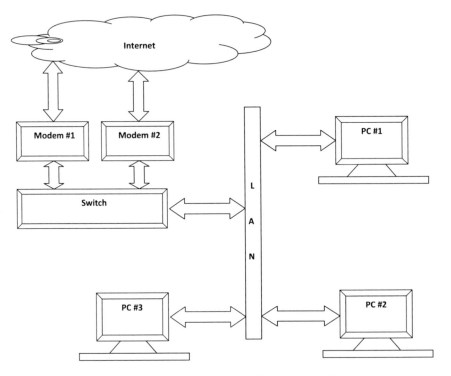

Fig. 6.1 Two internet connections to a switch.

6.2.2 Identifying non-critical Cloud-based Test Services

As mentioned earlier, it is imperative to access non-critical Cloud services from your premises for a period of at least 3 months before you can consider using a Cloud-based healthcare IT solution. Some of the Cloud-based services you should use for non-critical purposes are [1]–[3]:

1) Web based email such as yahoo mail, hotmail, gmail, etc.
2) Online Productivity tools such as Google Docs, Zoho, etc.
3) Web-based conferencing systems such as Gtalk, skype, etc.
4) Web-based data backup.

Over a three month period, it is necessary to actively use one or more of the above services and gather data about the Internet downtime and latency for your connections. There are tools that help you automatically track these numbers over a period of time [4].

6.2.3 Securing your Internal Network

Once you have an internet connection to your practice, it is necessary to safeguard your internal network and data. You should ask your IT consultant to do this, but it will typically involve:

1) Configuring your network to seamlessly crossover between two internet connections to ensure availability even if one connection goes down.
2) Installing security tools to filter traffic in and out of your network. Permission should only be allowed for data that is arriving from and going to approved domains.
3) Installing Antivirus software on computers.
4) Installing logging software to track network and site access from individual computers within the practice.
5) Installing security software to detect and flag the connection of any unauthorized media to any of the computers on the internal network.
6) Ensuring that Internet Browser settings are set to a level that provides the necessary level of security and at the same time allows the web services to run in the browser.
7) If your internal network is a wireless network, ensuring that it is secured and that access is protected.

The above exercise should put in place the infrastructure that is required to access and use Cloud services from within your premises. During this period, the following should be monitored and noted:

1) Incidence of viruses/security breaches. Indicates that your security products (firewalls/antiviruses/browser settings) are not properly configured
2) Network availability/downtime and the bandwidth and speed obtained on the network. If this is unsatisfactory, it means you either need to upgrade your internet plans or select another provider.

6.3 VENDOR SELECTION

There are many dozens of Healthcare IT solutions, and no matter what you are looking for, there is likely to be considerable choice for a solution to your requirements.

If your practice has more than 10 users of the IT system, it is recommended that you form a group of "super-users" from within your organization to conduct vendor evaluation and manage subsequent migration. The super-users should include physicians, nurse practitioners, and administrative staff members—essentially representatives of all types of users.

It can take up to several months to complete the process of identifying a vendor, getting internal systems organized and completing the transition to a Cloud-based system, depending on what a healthcare practice is looking for.

6.3.1 Best of breed products vs. products from a single vendor

As we saw in chapter 4, it takes several modules to create a comprehensive IT solution for a practice. This includes practice management, EMR, ePrescribing, billing module, and so on. In case of in-house IT solutions, it is often possible to obtain the best software for each requirement from a different vendor, and then integrate them so that they work together. The advantage of such a 'best-of-breed' approach is that you can get the best products for each purpose. In case of Cloud-based solutions, this is much harder to do. It is therefore necessary to look for a single Cloud-solution which includes modules for each function. Hence the process of evaluating a Cloud-based solution must consider every single aspect of the overall requirement.

6.3.2 Creating a Vendor Shortlist

STEP 1: The first step in identifying a Cloud IT solution is to create a shortlist of vendors that meet essential criteria. These are:

1) The solution needs to be certified by an approved certification agency.
2) The solution needs to be offered as a web-based service (either browser accessible or ASP model).

Because using a certified solution is essential, the first list of vendors is best drawn by researching the web-sites of the certification agencies for products that are certified. It is essential to ensure HIPAA & HITECH compliance. The certification needs to ensure that the product meets the Privacy and Security requirements of HIPAA, and also is able to meet the 'meaningful use' criteria defined in the HITECH act. Lastly, the product needs to be certified to meet the Interoperability requirements. Further information on certification is available in an appendix.

Lists of Healthcare IT solutions are also available at [5]–[7]. One can visit the websites of each of the listed products and determine the certification status of each of those.

Once the first list of certified products is determined, it can be ascertained which of these are available as web-based services from the information available on the websites of the product vendors.

STEP 2: The second criterion for narrowing the shortlist is the solution functionality. Since subscribing to 'best of breed' components and integrating them is not an option with Cloud-based products, it is necessary that the solution you choose meets all your requirements including any specific requirements of your specialty.

In case you are already using an in-house EMR system that you are happy with, it is a good idea to find out if the vendor already offers or has planned a release of a Cloud-based version. It is normally much easier to migrate from an in-house system to its Cloud-counterpart. Not only are you working with a single vendor, but the migration of data is likely to be easier, and the workflows are likely to be similar. This is likely to make it easier to adopt the Cloud version. If this is not the case, the best solution for your needs is to be determined from the list available.

The next step is to review the advertised functionality of the products on the list. This information is usually available on the vendor website. You should look for solutions which have the following attributes:

1) The Cloud-based solution should support your specialty. Every specialty has different requirements, and while some EMR solutions are generic, some of them are tailored for different specialties. You need to ensure upfront that a system is set up to support the workflows associated with your specialty, and comes pre-loaded with templates for the specialty.

2) The solution should include EMR, ePrescribing and Practice Management modules. These are the three key modules in any healthcare IT system and are necessary to demonstrate

'meaningful use' as defined in HITECH Act. These modules need to work seamlessly with each other as a part of an integrated system.

3) The solution should support a patient portal.

4) The solution should support Interoperability and should support HL7. Your solution will eventually need to work seamlessly with other systems, and therefore support for HL7 is necessary.

5) The solution should include a billing module. This could be a part of Practice Management in some solutions, but Medical Billing is a key feature for any practice.

The above step results in a short-list of solutions which are to be evaluated further.

6.3.3 Evaluating Cloud-based systems

Once a shortlist of products/vendors has been created as mentioned above, the next step is to evaluate the solutions on the shortlist to determine which of these is most suitable for your business. There are a number of factors based on which this evaluation is to be performed. These are discussed below. The best way to keep track of such an evaluation is to assign scores to each of the factors below, and then make a final decision keeping in mind the relative importance of each of these factors.

6.3.3.1 Functionality and Ease of Use

This is the first item to verify—whether the solution really includes the functionality you need to support your practice, and how easy it is to use. In many ways, this is the most important factor in the selection of a system. If the system you select is hard to use or requires substantial modification to your internal processes, adoption becomes that much harder, and you may eventually end up seeing far fewer patients than you do today. Secondly, the possibility of your staff making mistakes with such a solution is also higher. Therefore, the functionality and ease of use need to be evaluated in a systematic manner. Many Cloud-service providers offer limited-time free trial accounts. You should ask for such a trial account in order to actually exercise the functionality and verify that it meets your requirements. It is not enough to simply compare functionality based on marketing information supplied by vendors. It is necessary to actually exercise the features of all products and verify their operation for yourself. While doing this, the following pointers are helpful:

1) Identify the ten most frequently executed workflows in your practice. Workflows are 'operations' that you or your staff performs, and which you expect the software to handle for you. For example, a workflow may involve creating appointments for patients or following up on medical claims, or having previous charts of a particular patient available in a particular manner, etc. Then have the staff members who would be exercising those workflows try them on each of the shortlisted applications, to verify that they can indeed be supported easily. Some of these workflows would be specific to your specialty, so evaluating those workflows is necessary. The reason for focusing on only 10 common workflows is because typically there are a large number of operations you would perform with your IT system. It is impossible to exercise all of these in limited time. Creating a list of 10 most common workflows allows you to make sure that the tasks that you spend the most amount of time on are adequately evaluated. It is best to involve all the staff members (in a small practice) or at least several representatives across user groups (in larger practices) in the functional evaluation of applications. This ensures that the views of all users are taken into account while making a decision.

2) Make a list of features or functions that you consider critical in the system you acquire. (Note: This may be different from the list of ten *most frequent work-flows* mentioned above). For example, this could include items such as support for a particular data field in certain reports or support for directly importing readings from a particular type of medical device. You will need to ensure the presence of these features as a part of the functional evaluation.

Functional evaluation should be conducted at two levels—the presence of absence of a feature is the first level. Their ease of use is the second level. Even if two solutions support the same functionality, they may not be equally easy to use.

One way to conduct a functional evaluation is to assign a weightage to each function and then assign a numerical score based on the ability of a particular system to support that function (on a scale from 0 to 10 say). If you use the same list to evaluate each system, you are likely to have a numerical basis for comparing different systems at the end of your exercise.

There are a few key functionalities that an ambulatory practice must verify in an IT solution. Some of these are billing and accounts receivable, scheduling, in-house messaging, documentation of patient interactions, processing refill requests, reviewing and acting on lab results, managing external correspondence about patients, etc. These need to be on the list of functions to exercise in a system.

Functional evaluation is likely to be a time-consuming process, and your practice should set aside adequate time for completing functional evaluation of competing systems. You can also ask the vendor to provide you a demo of the product (this can be done over the web) specifically including a demo of the functionality and workflows you need. You can also ask to see a demo of your specialty templates.

6.3.3.2 *Vendor Business and Viability*

Cloud vendors have different types of business models. It is necessary to understand the nature of a solution vendor's business model for several reasons. Firstly, your Cloud-based Healthcare IT vendor going out of business is a nightmare scenario—something that can lead to substantial disruption to your practice, and potentially even loss of data. Secondly, it is in your interest to verify that your data remains private and secure and is not used in any manner you did not intend it to be used. Many Cloud startups use the advertising model to make revenues. Whether such advertising supported business model works for healthcare IT is not clear. It is necessary to find out how long the vendor has been in business, how many customers the vendor has and how long the specific product is being offered.

The financial viability of the Cloud provider is relevant to you because you trust the vendor with your data. For a public company, the financial figures are in the public domain. For a private company, it is important to estimate whether the business is viable. One way to estimate the revenues of the company is by estimating the number of users of the service. These figures are available on a number of third party sites such as compete.com, quantcast.com, alexa.com, etc. While none of these sites provide accurate numbers, they indicate trends, such as whether the company's user base is growing over a period of time or not. If the company offers free software, and a paid version, the number of customers of the paid version is likely to be a small fraction (10% is a reasonable estimate) of the total customers. Multiplying the number of customers by the subscription fee per user gives an idea of the revenues for the business. It is also a good idea to conduct web research on the vendor company, such as user-experience of other subscribers which can be found on blogs, analyst comments, product reviews, press-releases issued by the company, the investors in the company, etc.

The vendor should also be able to furnish a white paper or actual case studies based on current users of the system. It is useful if the case studies include information on the adoption process, and the ROI demonstrated by the vendor solution.

6.3.3.3 Support and Training

It is necessary to ask the Cloud-provider about the nature of customer-support that is available. Many companies provide email/ e-messenger support. For a healthcare IT offering, it is very useful to have 24x7 technical support available over voice (phone call). In the remote event that the Cloud-based system is not available when you need it, you should be able to talk to a person at any time of day or night, 365 days a year, in order to get your problem resolved. Unless a company charges for its services, it would typically not be able to make such support available to their customers. Such voice-based support is also valuable during the initial few weeks of using the system, when your staff is unfamiliar with the functionality.

If you are using a trial account during evaluation phase, make sure you call up the technical support and evaluate the quality of support that is provided. While some companies do an excellent job of selling the service, not all of them provide an equally high quality of post-sales support.

Training for staff is necessary before they begin to use a new system. It is necessary for the vendor to make such training available for your staff. If the vendor has created training videos that are adequately detailed, these maybe sufficient for users to get started on the software. The vendor also needs to provide the additional option of on-site training for a fee.

6.3.3.4 Cost of ownership

The total cost of using a Cloud-based service has several components to it. We have compared the cost of a Cloud-based service to the cost of an in-house system in chapter 3. Here we will address the task of comparing the costs of two Cloud-based services. The various components of the costs involved are:

1) Subscription fees. The subscription plans may differ across providers. For example, one provider may charge per-user-per-month, another provider may charge on the basis of storage space used and yet another provider may charge a flat annual fee. You will need to estimate your usage (number of users, data, etc.) and compute the cost of subscription fees for a year for all providers in order to make a fair comparison.

2) Training & Support costs. Training is usually charged separately, and the way it is charged differs from provider to provider. You will need to verify the kind of training that is available and the price at which it is available. Similarly, it is possible that a basic support plan is free, while higher levels of support are charged additionally. The cost of training and support needs to be determined for each provider and factored into the comparison.

3) Compliance costs (for HIPAA/HITECH). While it is necessary to use a certified product, there is additional responsibility on providers to ensure full compliance with HIPAA in ways that go beyond simply using certified software. Some of these responsibilities have been explained in an earlier chapter. It is necessary to estimate the cost of compliance for each of the provider solutions.

4) Conversion costs. Your practice may need to occasionally convert legacy paper based documents to the electronic form. You may have to get it done from your Cloud provider or an approved

partner or a third party service. It is necessary to determine the cost of such conversion of legacy data from each vendor.

It is not necessary that one should select the lowest cost vendor, but it is essential to get an idea of the costs prior to signing up for a service.

6.3.3.5 Data Storage

It is necessary to obtain clarity on the data storage practices of a Cloud service provider before subscribing to the service. We have seen in an earlier chapter the multiple security risks associated with data storage. Some of the questions to ask the provider include:

1) What is the location of the actual storage of data (country/ jurisdiction)
2) Does the provider have a system for remote backup? How frequently does the provider backup the data and where?
3) What are the policies around providing you a copy of your data? In what format is this data delivered? How long is legacy data stored? Can you obtain a date-wise snapshot of your data?
4) Will you have access to the data if the provider goes out of business?
5) What are the data security policies followed by the Cloud provider and have these been audited by a third party?

6.3.3.6 Infrastructure Security

It is a good practice for Cloud providers to conduct a Security Audit of their infrastructure from a third party and obtain certificate of security compliance. Security involves many facets. Some of these have been covered in an earlier chapter, and many issues dealing with security are deeply technical issues which cannot be reasonably evaluated by medical practitioners. Hence a third-party certificate of security audit provides valuable confirmation that the service provider's infrastructure is indeed robust.

6.3.3.7 Historical Outage Time

Outages are of two types—scheduled outages and unscheduled outages. Every Cloud provider needs to upgrade the service from time to time. Upgrades are necessary when technical issues ('bugs') in the system are fixed or when a new software release is ready. Upgrades are also necessary when new functionality or features are added to the software. The upgrade process will result in the service being unavailable for a short duration of time. This is known as a scheduled outage. It is possible that scheduled outages are planned once every week or even more frequently if the service is evolving.

The second types of outages are unscheduled outages, which refers to circumstances when the service becomes unavailable unintentionally. This could be a result of components within the system failing ('crashing')—a result of a hardware failure or a software flaw in the system. It could also result due to loss of connectivity at the service provider's Datacentre.

Several Cloud providers share details of their historical outage times—both scheduled and unscheduled.

6.3.3.8 User Agreements, Jurisdiction

Every Cloud Vendor has a user agreement that is to be agreed to by users of the service. It is necessary to read this User agreement carefully before subscribing to a Cloud service. User agreements are often complex; written by lawyers and intended to be read by lawyers. From a user view point though, it is best if these agreements are simple and unambiguous. User agreements need to be read with particular attention to the following points:

1) The jurisdiction under which the agreement is made. This tells you what sort of legal recourse you have should any dispute arise, and your ability to enforce the contract. This also defines the local laws that the provider needs to comply with.
2) The clauses pertaining to ownership of your data. Ideally, the ownership of your data should reside with you alone, and the Cloud vendor should undertake not to share it with any other party for any reason whatsoever.
3) Clauses pertaining to privacy and security of data. The Cloud vendor should undertake to make best efforts to ensure the security and privacy of your data, and comply with standards for data privacy and security as laid down in law. The agreement should also specify if and when your data will be destroyed after you cease to be a customer.

4) 'Service Level' clauses that define the benchmarks for system availability, support availability and so on and the recourse if these service benchmarks are not met.

5) Business Associate Agreement. The HIPAA defines anyone providing a service to a healthcare provider or having access to healthcare data as a 'Business Associate'. There are templates for Business Associate Agreements, which a Cloud Provider should be willing to enter into.

6.3.3.9 Patient Portal

The patient portal (a site from where your patients can login and access their medical records) is a required feature of Healthcare IT solutions. The Cloud-based system should have a patient portal as a part of its overall offering and provide patients the ability to login to the portal to view their medical records. The portal should also provide patients the ability to export their healthcare records in a standard format so that they can be imported into a PHR of the patient's choice. Lastly, the portal should support the ability to email any data.

6.3.3.10 User Authentication

For the purpose of added security it is useful if the access to the Cloud system is based on two 'factors' and not just a single password alone. The second authentication option (in addition to passwords) can be a hardware device such as a smart card (swiped into a smart card reader connected to your PC in order to enable access) or a hardware dongle connecting to the PC, etc. This ensures that someone who wants to access your account would not only need to know your password but also have access to the card/dongle.

There are other Identity verification schemes that are offered that ensure that the person accessing a site is who he/she claims to be.

It is also possible for Cloud service providers to restrict access to your account only from specific IP addresses. This ensures that only the PCs within your office can be used to access the Cloud service.

Incorporation of such features—'two factor authentication', ID verification, etc into cloud-solutions adds a further layer of security beyond what is offered by a password alone.

6.3.3.11 User Access Levels

There are normally different types of users of an IT system within a practice. This includes physicians, nurse practitioners, administrative staff, etc. HIPAA requires data access on an 'as-required' basis, which means that staff members who do not use healthcare data should not have access to it. One question to ask the provider is whether the IT system supports multiple 'user access levels' so that there is differentiation between the data is displayed at each level.

The practice needs to subsequently decide what access level to provide to each of its members.

6.3.3.12 Breach Notification

HIPAA lays down guidelines for notifying the patient and other agencies when private healthcare data about the patient is disclosed to an unauthorized entity. This is called 'Breach Notification' as discussed in detail in an earlier chapter. The Cloud provider needs to have systems in place for detecting such breaches and making the appropriate notifications when such a breach is detected. This should be a part of Business Associate Contract.

6.3.3.13 Subscriber References

Before signing up with any Cloud service you need to obtain at least 3 references of subscribers who are customers of the vendor and already using the Cloud-based system. It is best to seek references from practices that are of the same size as yours and work in the same specialty. If the reference subscribers have been using the system for more than 6 months, they typically have had an opportunity to use the various features of the system and form an opinion on usability of the system as well as the quality of service offered by the vendor. You should gather the following information from these references.

1) The uptime of the service. How frequently (if at all) was the service unavailable?

2) Ease of adoption. How easy was it to start using the system? Was there adequate training material available? How long did it take your practice to fully transition to using the system?

3) What sort of Internet connection speeds are needed for using the system?

4) Does the system work as advertised in terms of the features and functionality?

5) Are there any other issues with the system?

6.3.3.14 Other Security Features

It is desirable that the Cloud-based system has other additional security features. These include:

1) The application should time out (log itself out) if there is no activity for more than a certain amount of time. Imagine a situation where a staff member is working with patient health information on screen, and suddenly has to leave his desk for a few minutes. In such situations it is easy for the staff member to forget to log off from the system. This can result in a potential privacy breach if the information on screen is viewed by someone not authorized to do so. An even worse situation is when an unauthorized person uses the unattended terminal to access information about other patients. This danger can be mitigated to a certain extent by the requirement that the system log itself out automatically if there is no activity for a certain period of time. It is therefore useful if the system logs itself off after a period of inactivity.

2) The system should ensure that passwords created by users are of adequate strength and are changed at regular intervals. There is usually a tendency to choose simple passwords that are liable to be guessed or hacked. Passwords with combination of alpha-numeric and special characters are more suitable. Secondly, using the same password for a long period of time is not ideal. The system should therefore prompt all users to change their passwords every few months.

3) Some systems only communicate the login information over HTTPS and the rest of the data is sent over HTTP. However, it is necessary that all healthcare data and not just the username/

password be communicated over secure protocol (HTTPS). This ensures that no data can be intercepted and read over communication channels.

6.3.3.15 Customizability of Workflows

In some products, the workflows can be customized to your requirements. If the system meets your requirements as-is, there may not appear an immediate need for such customization. However, no Cloud vendor can exactly match the internal policies and procedures of your practice. Hence it is helpful to procure a product which can be modified or customized to your requirements. Customization may pertain to things such as the ability to define data fields in specific forms, the rules and limits for values in data fields, the sequence in which screens are displayed, the information displayed in printed reports, ability to modify practice management workflows, modify billing and audit practices, and so on. While too much customization is not a good thing, a certain amount of flexibility that allows users to modify the software to suit their requirements is a desirable feature of a Cloud-based application.

6.3.4 Secondary Criteria

In this section we will cover certain secondary criteria that impact your choice of a Cloud service solution. These are 'secondary' in the sense that they are relatively less important than the criteria covered in the earlier section.

6.3.4.1 Ability to export data to standard PHR (Personal Health Record Systems)

Not only is it necessary that the Cloud system comply with Interoperability requirements and conform with the standards specified therein, it is also useful if the system can export data to commonly used PHR systems such as Google Health or Microsoft HealthVault. This is in order to ensure that patients who need to obtain information from your system and maintain it in their PHR accounts can easily do so. There are many dozens of PHR systems and it is impractical to verify compatibility with each of them. However, it is a good idea to verify compatibility with atleast a couple of commonly used ones.

6.3.4.2 User Logs, Statistics

The Cloud provider needs to make available detailed usage logs of your organization on a periodic basis. Such logs would include information about:

1) Logins made by each user—login and log out time & date
2) IP address from which each login by each user was done
3) Patients whose records were touched during each login
4) Total data storage requirements of your organization
5) Total data traffic for the month till-date for your organization
6) Unsuccessful login attempts into accounts of your organization.

6.3.4.3 Digitizing Legacy Data

In case you are moving to a Cloud-based provider, it is likely that you have legacy data which you want to integrate/upload into the Cloud-based system. There are two possibilities. If you are already using an in-house Healthcare IT system, your legacy data is in electronic form and integrating it involves reformatting the legacy electronic data so that it can be read into your new Cloud-based system. For this purpose the Cloud-based system needs to either publish the format in which the system can read in data or provide such a service to prospective customers. In the first cast, i.e., when input data format is published, your practice may need to reformat legacy data so that it can be read into the Cloud-based system. In the second case, it is necessary to determine the cost of contracting the service for data migration.

Another scenario involves digitizing older paper based records. There are several consulting firms that offer medical record digitization services. It is not enough to simply scan the older records. If the information in them has to be entered into the Cloud-based system, it is necessary to extract information from the paper records and format it in a manner such that it can be read into the Cloud-based system.

6.3.4.4 Availability of an API

An API—Application Programming Interface is a set of functions that can be invoked to access and manipulate data stored in the

Cloud-based system. If a Cloud provider publishes such an API for the system, it results in several benefits for the customer:

1) Such an API is likely to permit the import of legacy data into the system as discussed in the earlier section.

2) Availability of API allows you to perform other data operations which may not be supported by the vendor's system itself. For example, the API could possibly allow you to backup your data on a third party backup service such that it is accessible to you independent of your Cloud service provider. Another example is of the API being used by you to generate custom reports that your practice requires.

3) If an API is published and known, it is likely that 'third-party' applications would be developed for the system by other developers. This only increases the functionality and applications that are available to you. Larger companies such as Google Health and Microsoft HealthVault have already published API for their respective systems and this has resulted in spawning large communities of third party developers and applications.

6.3.4.5 eVisits

eVisits are a desirable feature of any Cloud-based system. eVisits, as discussed in an earlier chapter pertain to the patient's ability to reach and consult healthcare practitioners electronically. This includes means such as sending emails to physicians, being able to initiate and engage in electronic 'chat' with a physician or nurse practitioner at any time, or even being able to engage in a video chat with a practitioner. This functionality is easy to integrate into Cloud-based systems and is a useful feature to have.

6.3.4.6 Data Exchange with Local Hospital

Before subscribing to a service, it is useful to ensure that the service you select can exchange data with the local hospital at which your patients are likely to be admitted for surgeries or other procedures. This again, pertains to interoperability of your Cloud-based service with the IT system that the local hospital is using. Such interoperability means that you can import a patient's data from the hospital's IT system into the solution you are using, and vice versa.

6.3.4.7 Ability to Connect Devices

Measuring devices are now available which connect directly into the EMR system of the practice. This ensures higher accuracy of the stored data, and also saves valuable time. For e.g., Microsoft HealthVault supports interfacing with a large number of devices such that their readings can be directly stored in the PHR. Similarly, it is possible to directly upload device measurements into some Cloud-based EMR solutions.

6.3.4.8 Search Capability

The ability to search records based on keywords is a useful feature than can save a practitioner considerable time. Having basic and advanced search capability within the system is therefore a plus.

6.3.4.9 Number of releases made in the past year

The number of releases of a product within a prior one-year period is indicative of how quickly the product is evolving. Too many releases being made too quickly may indicate a responsive vendor, although it may also indicate a product that is not yet mature.

6.3.4.10 Client Access Software

Many Cloud services allow access using any standard Internet Browser. Some Cloud services may require you to download a 'plugin' for your browser. (A 'plugin' is a piece of software that runs within the browser and enables you to access the Cloud service.) For other Cloud-based services, you may need a remote access or a VPN client to be installed on your PC.

It is necessary to know upfront whether the service is plain browser accessible or requires such plugins or other software installed on your PC. If such software is required, it may impact your ability to access the service from a mobile device. Remote access/VPN software does not work well from all mobile/handheld systems and plugins may not work on all mobile browsers. If mobile access is important for you, it is necessary to ensure that the system is accessible from your particular mobile browser.

6.3.4.11 Support for PQRI Automation

PQRI (Physician Quality Reporting Initiative) is being increasingly supported by CMS with financial incentives. Those physicians who want to follow the PQRI guidelines will need to generate and report data on a variety of quality-measures. Such physicians need to ensure that the system they choose provides automation and support for generating the documentation and reports required for PQRI compliance.

6.3.4.12 Support for voice and handwriting recognition

Speech recognition technology is being widely used in healthcare because it leads to an enormous saving of time for clinical staff. Similarly handwriting recognition technology is gaining acceptance due to the proliferation of hand-held/mobile devices such as tablets and palm-top computers. Ability of a solution to integrate handwriting recognition and voice recognition systems is therefore a very desirable feature to have in a Cloud-based solution.

6.4 ADOPTING A CLOUD SERVICE

By the time you have completed the stages outlined in the earlier sections of this chapter, you would have done the following:

1) Ensured that the infrastructure within your practice is setup in order to be able to access and use a Cloud-based solution. This includes computers for staff, networking infrastructure (either Ethernet or wireless) that connects the computers within the practice and redundant internet connections for external connectivity.
2) Installed appropriate security systems in order to guard against external attacks on your infrastructure or against malware entering your internal network.
3) Obtained experience in using non-critical Cloud-based applications using the infrastructure
4) Conducted an evaluation of various Cloud-based solutions and identified the solution that you intend to migrate to.

Migrating to any new IT system has to be carefully planned and it is no different with Cloud-based systems. The migration plan is best developed in conjunction with the solution vendor. In this section we will cover some generic guidelines for this migration.

The migration plan should include the following:

1) A clear definition of roles and responsibilities for people within the practice.
2) Training schedule for all users of the system
3) Plan for migrating legacy data
4) Plan for sequence in which modules will be adopted/migrated.
5) Timelines for completing the process of migration.

6.4.1 Training

The training material to be obtained from the Cloud-vendor usually includes:

1) Online user manuals
2) Training videos/demo recordings showing step by step usage of the system
3) User training exercises.

Initial training on every single aspect of the system is unrealistic. However the initial training should cover the following aspects:

1) Training on the 10 most common workflows of your practice
2) Training on exercising the critical functionality (the list used during vendor evaluation)
3) Training on Privacy and Security features of the system
4) Training on assisting your patients to obtain their data from the system (via the patient portal)
5) Training on backing up all your data from the service provider to secondary storage on your premises or with another Cloud provider.

Additionally, as mentioned in an earlier chapter, training the staff on relevant provisions of HIPAA/HITECH is also necessary.

6.4.2 Reorganizing internal processes and workflows and documenting the modifications

It is possible that the IT system you select supports all the workflows and functionality you need, but requires modification to the internal procedures presently employed within your practice. If customizing the software is not possible, it means a reorganization of your internal processes is necessary so that they are aligned with your IT system. Some of these changes may also be dictated by the enhanced requirements around security and privacy of healthcare information, and the other audit and reporting obligations placed upon healthcare providers by HIPAA. This presents an opportunity to review and optimize your internal processes so that they are streamlined or made more efficient.

This is an important step in adoption of a Cloud-based system —the aligning of procedures and practices within your clinic to the workflows supported by the software. The information on modified internal workflows needs to be documented and included within the training materials so that it is readily accessible to the clinical and non-clinical users of the system.

6.4.3 Creating Policies, Documentation, Notice of Privacy, Risk Assessment, Audit mechanisms

The documentation required by HIPAA has been covered in an earlier chapter. This needs to be put in place during the process of adopting the Cloud-service.

6.4.4 Migrating Legacy Data

Legacy data refers to older medical records of patients which are probably in paper form or in a different electronic format. This legacy data needs to be accessible to the physician at the time of meeting the patient. Traditionally, an administrative staff member retrieves the paper records (charts) and keeps them ready for the patient's meeting with the physician. If the physician is using a Cloud-based system, the legacy data needs to be ported into the Cloud-based system so that it is accessible to the physician during the patient meeting.

There are several ways to approach the task of porting legacy data. Some practices take up this task upfront, i.e., they first import all legacy data into the Cloud-based system before beginning to use the system. This requires the practice to contract with either the Cloud-provider or a third-party service to digitize all the patient records and enter them into the Cloud-based system. This approach is convenient for physicians and care providers, because all data is available in the electronic system at the time they begin to use it. On the other hand, this approach entails significant upfront expenses associated with digitizing all paper records. It can also delay the adoption of the Cloud-based system. The other drawback to doing all digitization upfront is that you also pay to convert the data of patients who may never come to meet you.

The second approach which some practices adopt is to convert the data of patients after they seek an appointment. In other words, legacy data is entered into the Cloud-based system just before it is required by the physician. In this approach the conversion effort is distributed over a longer period of time rather than being undertaken upfront. It also means that the data is only converted for patients who actually need to see the physician.

A third approach is a hybrid approach—which is to convert the legacy data of only 'active' patients upfront. This means that the data of the patients who visit frequently is converted upfront, and the data of remaining patients is converted on as as-required basis. For example, records of 20% of patients who visit the practice most frequently can be digitized initially and for other patients data is converted as and when they seek appointment.

The practice needs to decide on and adopt one of these approaches for porting data to the Cloud-based system.

6.4.5 Sequence for transitioning modules

If you are subscribing to an integrated solution that includes several modules such as EMR, Practice Management, ePrescribing, and so on, there is always a question of whether to adopt the entire solution simultaneously or adopt modules one by one. Both approaches have their pros and cons. Based on experience of several practices that have performed such a transition, it is probably easier to transition few modules at a time rather than abruptly moving to the Cloud-based system entirely in one go. Although this draws out the transition process, it also minimizes the probability of errors and is easier for the users.

If your practice plans to adopt one module at a time, it is natural to ask the sequence in which the modules should be adopted. The following sequence is recommended, again based on the experience of practices that have performed such a transition:

1) *Practice Management.* Practice Management deals with the management of non-clinical aspects of a healthcare provider such as managing patient appointments, billing, and so on. It is not a very specialty-sensitive module. Its direct impact on physicians and nurse-practitioners is relatively less although it does impact the administrative staff. It is therefore a module that can be adopted before all others. Beginning with this module allows everyone to develop familiarity with Cloud-based systems and also provides more time for training.

2) *EMR System.* This is the most critical element of healthcare IT, and adopting this module can potentially take the longest time. Adopting it early allows practices to implement and operationalize security and privacy policies and processes. It also allows practices to put in place reporting and auditing mechanisms to demonstrate compliance with HIPAA and HITECH.

3) *ePrescribing.* This again is a module which is required to meet the requirements of the HITECH act. However it is a module that avoids significant productivity hit. Adopting it immediately after adopting EMR is useful from a point of view of HITECH compliance.

4) *Electronic Messaging, Document scanning, eVisits, Patient Portal, Lab data interfaces, Electronic Charting,* etc. These are the modules that are best handled towards the end. Out of these, eVisits and Electronic Charting are generally harder to adopt, and take substantial time.

6.4.6 Intermediate Phase of using both; paper/legacy system and Cloud-based system

One question that is often asked is whether a practice should make a clean break from the earlier system, i.e., entirely discontinue the use of earlier system and move over to a Cloud-based system one day, or, is it better to have a more gradual transition, wherein for a certain amount of time, both systems (earlier system as well as the new Cloud-based system) are used.

The first approach is risky, though if successfully implemented can lead to a much faster transition. It is risky because it is error prone. There is a higher chance that administration of healthcare can be impacted if system users are unable to efficiently and correctly use the new system immediately.

In the second approach, practices continue to use the old and new systems (both together) for a small amount of time say about 2–4 weeks. During this period, because two systems are being used, the overall efficiency is significantly impacted. Data needs to be duplicated at two different places. However, this is a safer approach because administration of healthcare is not impacted. A transition to a Cloud-based system is made after clinical and non-clinical staff is comfortable in their ability to use it exclusively. Practices that have followed this approach report up to 50% drop in the number of patients they can see within this period, and it should be accepted that physicians will be able to see much fewer patients during this intermediate stage.

6.4.7 Preparing for Meaningful Use targets

The practice needs to appoint a compliance officer whose responsibility it will be to ensure that the benchmarks for attaining the targets for 'meaningful use' are met. This includes goals for documentation, ePrescribing, reporting and so on. Attainment of these goals needs to be monitored on a periodic basis. These goals are covered in an appendix.

6.5 POST INSTALLATION

There are a number of steps a healthcare organization needs to take periodically after commencing the use of a Cloud service. Some of these are:

1) Making sure that the audit, documentation and reporting requirements of HIPAA/HITECH are complied with from time to time.

2) Ensuring that the security tools used in the practice are regularly upgraded. This includes installing upgrades to anti-virus and firewall software when such upgrades are available. It also includes installing browser patches as they become available.

3) Upgrading the internet connection bandwidth as your usage increases.

4) Periodically backing up data to another provider or to another location.

5) Providing training to your staff on new features of the software as they are released.

REFERENCES

[1] http://www.googledocs.com

[2] http://www.zoho.com

[3] http://www.skype.com

[4] http://www.cloudforhit.com

[5] http://www.healthcare-informatics.com/ME2/dirsect.asp?sid=3FD926E0A
    2884506947FD7451869716C&nm=The+2010+HCI+100+List

[6] http://www.revenuexl.com/emr-vendor-selection/

[7] http://www.medicexchange.com/EMR-Products-Systems.html

SECTION III

TOPICS IN HEALTHCARE IT

CHAPTER 7

Interoperability

Several times in this book so far, we have mentioned that one of the key benefits of adopting electronic medical records (EMR) is the subsequent ability to exchange EMR data among various care providers. Why is it necessary for the systems used by various healthcare players (providers, payers, labs, etc.) to be able to communicate with each other electronically? How can such seamless communication be achieved? How can physicians and care givers benefit from such information transfer?

The subject of this chapter is Interoperability—which refers to the ability of healthcare IT systems to securely communicate healthcare data with each other. We will also see why Cloud-based systems are inherently better suited when it comes to adopting emerging interoperability standards.

7.1 NEED FOR INTEROPERABILITY

1) In many countries including the US, people have a choice of providers from whom they can obtain their healthcare. When a large number of providers are private entities, people base their choice on factors such as quality of care provided, nearness to home/place of work, anecdotal information or feedback from relatives and friends, and so on. Most people, including Americans obtain healthcare from more than one provider. They visit family physicians, or specialists if need arises. They go to hospitals for surgeries and other procedures. Laboratory tests, Radiology tests, etc are done at specialized labs, and medicines are procured against prescriptions from pharmacies. In addition,

there are emergency centers, work-site clinics, school clinics, or public health centers where people may access healthcare. Healthcare information needs to be sent to payers, insurers and even public health bodies. Lastly, some organizations may outsource some of their care to other providers from time to time for a variety of reasons. This means that healthcare records for a single person are generated at many different locations at different times. It is in the interest of patients if their healthcare records are consolidated into a single repository, and these consolidated records are made available at the place and time when patients need medical care.

2) People frequently change their primary healthcare provider. This is for a number of reasons such as because they relocate, because they change their insurance company or employer or simply feel they can obtain better healthcare elsewhere. In such situations, all healthcare records with the earlier provider need to be transferred to the new provider for continued care.

3) When people are travelling and need to access healthcare, they are most likely to visit a provider who they have never been to before. This is most likely to happen in emergent situations. It is necessary in such a situation that the person's historical medical records be available to the attending physician before medical care is administered.

The above three scenarios highlight the necessity of being able to transfer or exchange healthcare data. Because there does not exist a robust national infrastructure for exchanging healthcare records today, this exchange takes the form of documents being faxed between organizations, or information being shared by voice over phone. These information transfer mechanisms are not ideal. When documents are sent over fax, it is possible that these documents are handled by people who do not have the need to access them. Medical information being dictated over phone can also result in violation of the patient's privacy. Moreover, information could be lost or misunderstood when communicated over phone. Furthermore, the time spent in locating and sending medical information over a phone or fax is significant. If needed medical documents are not immediately available at the point of care, it compromises the physician's ability to make decisions.

There is a clear need for creating an infrastructure that allows healthcare information to be exchanged rapidly and securely among various providers and entities in the healthcare industry. The goal of such a system is to make a person's healthcare information available at any time or place where it is required for provision of healthcare services. This data exchange is in the interest of the physicians as well. If physicians have access to up-to-date patient history, they can obviously administer better care rather than making critical decisions on the basis of incomplete facts.

If the goal of medical information always being available at the point of care is to be realized, it would require that the hundreds of thousands of care providers be able to exchange information and communicate medical records seamlessly, while simultaneously adhering to the privacy and security guidelines as laid down in HIPAA. This is a significant problem—there are more than 600,000 physicians in the US, almost half of whom are not affiliated with large hospitals. There are probably around 25,000 provider organizations such as hospitals, clinics and nursing facilities.

In order to address this significant problem of connecting such a large number of providers, the office of health and Human Services (HHS) established the Nationwide Health Information Network (NHIN), which is a set of standards and policies that enable the exchange of health information among diverse entities within the healthcare system securely over public network. The NHIN seeks to achieve Interoperability by defining a common set of protocols and standards for information exchange. In some communities/states/ districts, Healthcare Information Exchanges (HIE) or Regional Health Information Organizations (RHIO) have emerged, with an objective of connecting all providers within a group with each other and allow sharing and exchange of data where and when required.

An equivalent example exists in the financial domain, where a similar challenge existed—that of connecting hundreds of thousands of merchants so that they could receive credit card payments. The subsequent proliferation of Credit card processing terminals happened because merchants saw value in being connected—that they could now offer better service to their customers. A similar proliferation of connected healthcare systems is envisaged in the future.

7.2 WHAT IS INTEROPERABILITY?

Interoperability between systems refers to their ability to exchange information in a manner so that it is interpreted and understood in the same way by the sender and the receiver. In the case of Healthcare IT, Interoperability refers to the ability of different healthcare IT systems to exchange healthcare related information so that it is understood exactly the same way by all systems and the physicians who access those systems.

[1] provides a detailed overview of how the definition of Interoperability evolved, and its various aspects in the context of healthcare.

7.2.1 Types of interoperability

If two systems are to be made 'interoperable', it usually involves creating common mechanisms at multiple levels. Firstly, the systems need to be able to communicate with each other at a network level, in the sense that they should be electronically connected and be able to send and receive 'bit-streams' from each other. Secondly, it is necessary that the bit streams be processed in the same way by the systems on both sides. Thirdly, it is necessary that the information contained within the bit-streams be interpreted & understood in the same way by the human staff on both sides.

Overall Interoperability encompasses the following:

7.2.1.1 Technical Interoperability

Technical interoperability refers to the most basic, infrastructure-level interoperability between two systems. In other words, it refers to their ability to exchange sequences of bytes with each other ('Bytes' is used as a unit of information, one byte refers to a sequence of 8 'bits'. Each bit can have the value 0 or 1). Technical interoperability assures the existence of an electronic communication channel between two systems over which digital signals can be sent from one system to another. This also means that each system has a transmitter that can send a sequence of bytes and a receiver that can receive a sequence of bytes. Note that in most cases, the 'communication channel' is not necessarily direct, but can involve intermediate communication hubs. For example, when two systems are connected over the internet, the digital traffic between them involves passage through several internet gateways. The 'transmitter' and 'receiver' referred to earlier are simply the modems that are used to access the Internet which are usually a component of the IT infrastructure of any provider. Ensuring Technical Interoperability in Healthcare IT therefore requires that Healthcare IT systems be connected to a common communication infrastructure such as the Internet and be able to send and receive information to each other.

The focus of technical interoperability is on the ability to send and receive data. It is not concerned with the actual interpretation of the data. As mentioned in [2], Technical Interoperability neutralizes the effect of distance.

7.2.1.2 Semantic Interoperability

Semantic Interoperability refers to the ability of two systems to interpret byte-sequences in exactly the same way. Communicated byte-sequences have no value if they are not understood in an identical manner by the sender and the recipient. It is Semantic Interoperability that allows exchanged byte-sequences to be treated as actual 'information'.

Semantic Interoperability itself has many facets. For example, it requires that the sender and receiver follow a common protocol and a common format for sending information. A protocol refers to the manner in which information exchange will happen—the sequence of messages to be exchanged for a particular objective. A format on the other hand dictates the meaning of each byte within a single message. These common protocols and formats need to be agreed upon in advance, so that the byte sequences that are sent by the sending system are compliant with the agreed protocol and format. This in turn allows the receiving system to interpret the data in a pre-agreed manner. One common format for data exchange that is widely used is the XML format. XML stands for "Extensible Markup Language".

The sender and receiver not only need to pre-agree on a common protocol and a common message format, but they also need to speak the same language. In other words they need to share a common terminology & grammar. Particularly when non-numerical information is to be exchanged, it is essential that the same terminology be used to describe medical conditions, treatments, medications etc by both the sender and the receiver. If information received is to be processed by a machine, it is essential that the sender use a language which the processing machine at the receiver end can understand. This is only possible by defining a common vocabulary or a common set of codes that are accepted and understood by everybody. Semantic interoperability communicates meaning. It is not only important in situations when received information is processed by humans, but also in situations where the received information is processed by machines.

When both types of interoperability (technical and semantic) are present, the systems are fully interoperable, and the physicians attending to the patient at the hospital are able to obtain and then understand exactly the medical history of the patient. Full interoperability enhances the chances of proper care being administered, consequently improving healthcare outcomes. Additionally, the received information can also be integrated into the recipient's IT system for future reference or use.

In [1], the authors take a closer look at levels of Interoperability within each type. For example, when it comes to Technical Interoperability, the simplest case is a unidirectional transmission of a message over a network and its correct receipt. There are more complex communication protocols that result in structured information exchange. Similarly, sending a scan of a handwritten document containing free text in English, readable by a human is a simple case of Semantic Interoperability. On the other hand, digital information (searchable, editable) containing codes from International Classification of Diseases (ICD-9) or SNOMED (Standardized Nomenclature of Medicine) is an example of a complex semantic interoperability.

7.3 HEALTHCARE INFORMATION EXCHANGES AND REGIONAL HEALTH INFORMATION ORGANIZATIONS

In the earlier sections, we covered the definition of Interoperability, the need for Interoperability and its various aspects. In this section, we will cover the operational aspects—How is Interoperability sought to be achieved at a regional and even national level.

Information exchange among healthcare providers is sought to be achieved via an infrastructure that relies on intermediaries, known as Health Information Exchanges (HIE) or Regional Health Information Organizations (RHIO). The two terms are often used interchangeably. Their purpose is the systematic exchange of up-to-date healthcare information among healthcare providers so that the information is always available at the point of care. They are intermediaries, which perform two functions—firstly they receive and store healthcare data and secondly they forward healthcare data to the location where it is needed. As far as their storage function is concerned, they act as information repositories—where patient medical records gathered from multiple healthcare providers—hospitals, clinics, office physicians, laboratories, etc are stored and maintained. As far as their 'information forwarding' role is concerned, healthcare providers are in a position to seek the latest records for patients from them.

This means that:

1) Care providers are connected to HIEs. HIEs are set up as Information Hubs, linking numerous healthcare providers (the spokes connected to the hub).

2) When Care Providers update medical records of a patient, the modified information is communicated to the HIE. The HIE updates the records of that patient with the modification in its database.

3) Care providers access medical records in an HIE when care needs to be administered. When a Healthcare provider encounters a patient whose prior EHR is not available on the provider's internal records (such as a new patient) the provider can seek the prior medical records of the patient from the HIE.

To summarize, the HIE acts as a 'switchboard' which routes patient records, medical histories, test results, administrative and financial information between physician practices, hospitals, clinics, laboratories, payers and essentially all the entities in the healthcare ecosystem.

7.3.1 The advantage of HIEs and RHIOs

Figure 7.1 shows a number of healthcare providers in an area that exchange healthcare information among themselves directly rather

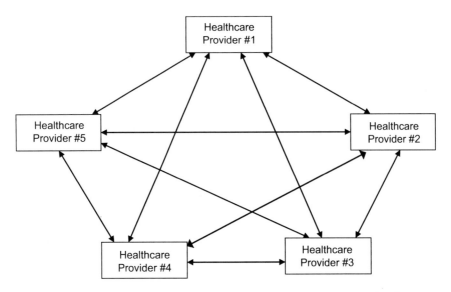

Fig. 7.1 Healthcare Providers with direct connectivity among each other.

than going through an intermediary or a HIE. While it is technically possible for providers to exchange information directly, such an arrangement has several drawbacks:

1) Because each provider has to talk to every other provider, it results in a large number of interconnections—10 in the above case of 5 providers. This means each provider has to negotiate a communication protocol with every other provider, which is a significant logistical challenge.

2) The latest records of every patient have to be communicated to and maintained with each provider. Any time a provider provides care to a patient, the patient information update is communicated to every other provider. This is inefficient in terms of storage and bandwidth utilization.

3) Addition of more providers to the network is hard, because the new provider needs to communicate information to every other existing provider in the network—the size of the problem only grows as more and more providers join the network.

The setting up of an Information Intermediary results in a configuration as shown in Fig. 7.2, and resolves the problems mentioned above. In such an arrangement involving the intermediary:

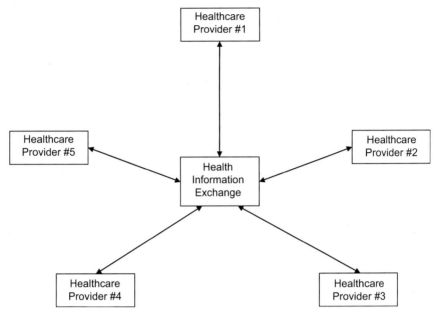

Fig. 7.2 Healthcare Providers connected via an HIE.

1) Each Provider only communicates with the Intermediary, i.e., one other entity. This means each provider has to ensure compliance with communication protocols of only one other entity, which is the exchange.

2) Latest information about patients needs to be communicated only to the exchange. Conversely, the latest information about any patient can be fetched from the exchange. Not only does this reduce the bandwidth requirements but also means that data storage happens in only one place.

3) Addition of more providers to the network is easier—they simply need to begin communicating with the exchange.

HIEs often store and exchange not only clinical data, but financial and administrative data as well. HIEs bring quality, efficiency, and savings to the process of exchanging healthcare information. This benefits everyone. Clinicians benefit because they have accurate, comprehensive and latest medical records of a patient available to them while providing care. Patients stand to benefit because availability of such information with the physician results in better care. One of the more significant benefits of this to the patient is that it often eliminates the need for repeating laboratory tests.

Health Information Exchanges are hence the preferred method for ensuring Interoperability among healthcare providers. Numerous HIEs are functioning in various geographies, and several of them have governmental support. Most have already resulted in substantial reduction of overall healthcare costs, and met the objective of providing better care. Examples of HIEs that are already operational include Michiana Health Information Network, Sushoo Health Information Exchange, Long Island Patient Information Exchange, Indiana Health Information Exchange, etc. The US Department of Health and Human Services has published a report [3] which outlines the progress of several Health Information Exchanges.

The eventual National Health Information Network (NHIN) which will be setup in the US will interconnect various HIEs, thereby ensuring Interoperability across the country. This is shown in Fig. 7.3.

From a technology perspective, HIEs need to be able to ensure reliable and secure transfer of information between themselves and the providers. They must also be able to ensure the reliable, secure archival of medical records. Healthcare Information Exchanges therefore focus on the areas of technology, interoperability, standards utilization, and business information systems.

Sample summary for one particular HIE is provided as an appendix.

7.4 AN EXAMPLE OF INTEROPERABILITY

As an example of Interoperability demonstrating the concepts discussed in earlier sections, consider a situation where a patient who normally obtains healthcare from his local community health centre is travelling to a different city. During the course of travel, the patient suffers a stroke and needs to be hospitalized immediately in a different city which is geographically remote from his usual local community health centre. Thankfully, the patient is carrying with him his Identification and Insurance information that enables his treatment to proceed immediately. The hospital now attending to the patient queries the Health Information Exchange for records of comprehensive medical history of the patient which will enable the attending physicians understand the prior medical history of the

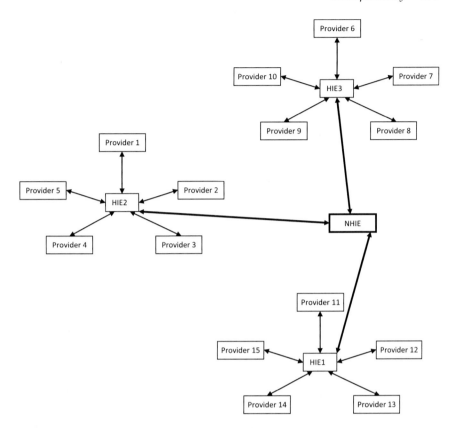

Fig. 7.3 National Health Information Exchange.

patient. The Health Information Exchange has the latest records of the patient because the community centre is linked to it, and stores its patient records with the HIE. The query from the hospital to the HIE and the response from the HIE to the hospital are electronic and happen over the Internet, rather than over a fax machine.

The ability to establish reliable two way communication, i.e., the ability of the hospital to query the HIE, and conversely the ability of the HIE to respond to the hospital over a shared communication infrastructure is a result of Technical Interoperability. The fact that the two are physically located at geographically distant locations is nullified by the fact that the two have technical interoperability thereby making information sharing feasible.

The data received from the HIE is not useful if it cannot be interpreted by the physicians attending to the patient. The sender and the receiver follow a common pre-agreed format to which the data conforms. Secondly, the information contained follows a common vocabulary, codes and semantic standards. If the data is so structured and uses a shared vocabulary, it can be unambiguously interpreted by the receiving physician, or even a machine that is suitably programmed.

Semantic Interoperability helps the understanding of data whose transportation is enabled by technical interoperability. The existence of HIEs ensures that the data can be quickly looked up, and the latest data becomes available at the point of care instantly.

7.5 INTEROPERABILITY STANDARD HL7

The existence of data communication standards is at the heart of Interoperability. Interoperability is possible because different providers and systems have embraced common standards for exchanging information. Several such common standards have emerged out of which HL7 is one [4]. Standards such as these are typically proposed by standard-making bodies which include experts and practitioners from different areas within that domain. HL7 is important because it is a standard that is supported by around 80% of healthcare IT systems in the US. In this section we will understand the evolution of this standard, the structure of its messages, and the type of information that can be communicated with this standard. It is useful for practitioners to know about HL7 because it helps them understand what exactly can be communicated by such standards.

7.5.1 What is HL7?

Health Level Seven International (HL7) is a not-for-profit organization which was founded in 1987. It is a Standards Developing Organization (one of several in the healthcare area) affiliated to American National Standards Institute (ANSI). Its vision is to create the best and most widely used standards in healthcare in order to improve care delivery. HL7 has created a comprehensive framework along with the required standards for the sharing and storage of electronic health information among multiple applications, devices and systems. HL7 is therefore a critical piece in the delivery of health services—not only clinical care but overall patient management as well. HL7 can be used to optimize process workflows, eliminate ambiguity and enhance knowledge transfer among healthcare providers, government agencies, payers, application vendors, and patients.

The HL7 organization has thousands of members which includes more than 90% of the Healthcare IT system vendors. Compliance with HL7 is therefore the quickest way to interface with most systems and applications available and installed in the industry today.

The name HL7 has its roots in the seven-layer communications model for Open Systems Interconnection (OSI) proposed by the International Organization for Standardization (ISO). The seven layers in this model are:

1) Physical Layer, which pertains to the connection between the communication entity and the communication medium

2) Data Link Layer which pertains to the error control between two nodes of the network.

3) Network Layer which pertains to how the information is routed on the network

4) Transport Layer which pertains to the end-to-end communication control

5) Session Layer which pertains to the problems that are not communication issues

6) Presentation Layer which pertains to the conversion of the information to formats which are usable

7) Application Layer which pertains to the provision of services to the applications.

The name Health Level 7 takes from the seventh layer (Application Layer) of the OSI model. HL7 primarily deals with how healthcare applications can interface with and communicate with each other.

7.5.2 HL7 Interoperability among Healthcare Applications

Healthcare domain is unique because of the sheer number of different entities involved in the overall business of providing healthcare. There are healthcare providers (such as hospitals, clinics, etc.), there are specialists with individual practices, there are payers and insurance companies, there are test laboratories (such as pathology labs, radiology centers), there are pharmacies, government agencies, software vendors, device manufacturers, and so on. Each of these entities is independent, and uses systems of its choice. If the entities in the healthcare space are operating within silos, the communication between two different vendor systems can only be done by customizing the two systems on the basis of a common interface standard between them. This is clearly not optimal, because it requires substantial investment of time and effort every time two systems have a need for communicating with one another. There are literally thousands IT systems and devices that deal with healthcare. Each of these systems or devices has information which it needs to communicate. The challenge of getting so many diverse systems to talk to each other is what makes a standard such as HL7 necessary.

HL7 was created in order to eliminate the problem of building custom interfaces on a case-by-case basis. It was created so that any healthcare system could exchange data with any other healthcare system. Finally, it was created to ensure that any applications created in the future would be able to communicate with the systems in use today. To summarize, HL7 was created in order to ensure information compatibility of all present and future healthcare IT systems.

Over 90% of the healthcare IT systems in the US today are compliant with HL7 standards, in other words, these are capable of communicating with each other via this common protocol. This includes clinical information systems, clinical applications including EMR systems, ePrescription systems and pharmacy systems, systems used by payers and insurance companies, devices that can now directly input data into clinical information systems, practice management systems in hospitals and clinics and IT systems being run by government bodies for gathering data. In other words, HL7 has emerged as the de facto standard for all of the data exchange needs in the healthcare industry.

HL7 evolved over a period of time, with many different individuals, organizations and agencies contributing to its evolution voluntarily, including clinical specialists, device manufacturers, software vendors and policy specialists. The standard has evolved in response to actual data interface challenges observed by practitioners. Over a period of time, points of data exchange have been identified, along with the nature of information that needs to be exchanged at those points. The standard has evolved to support the particular exchange required at the identified point.

Because it has its genesis in the practical data exchange problems faced in the industry, HL7 is now well-suited to address the challenge of interoperability in healthcare.

7.5.3 HL7 Standards

HL7 has contributed a number of standards so far, pertaining to various aspects of healthcare Information exchange [4]. These are:

Version 2.x Messaging Standard

This standard is also known as the "Application Protocol for Electronic Data Exchange in Healthcare Environments" and is a specification for automated (computerized) sending and receiving of transactions arranged by domain. Each transaction may involve sending and receiving of messages more than once.

Version 3 Messaging Standard

This standard is an interoperability specification for transactions that are derived from the HL7 V3 Foundation models and vocabulary and are also used to define communications transmitted and received by computer systems domain-wise. This standard incorporates the concepts of message wrappers, sequential interactions, and model-based message payloads.

Version 3 Rules/GELLO

GELLO is a standard expression language for decision support. The syntax of the GELLO language is based on the Object Constraint Language (OCL). OCL was developed by the Object Management Group (OMG) as a constraint and query language for UML class models. Given that it is based on UML, GELLO was designed to leverage the semantics of HL7 Version 3 Reference Information Model (RIM) and associated Refined Message Information Models (R-MIMs), in combination with HL7 Vocabulary and Data Types, for clinical decision support.

Arden Syntax

Arden is a "rules syntax" specification that allows rules to be individually published independently of a computer system and subsequently imported into computer systems for healthcare use. Arden implementation guides are published in a modular format by content providers, a guide for each rule.

CCOW/Visual Integration

Visual Integration Messages are an interoperability specification for visual integration of applications that allows users to experience an integrated computer-user session on the desktop. Clinical Context Object Workgroup is an interoperability specification as well. Messages are specified that flow between presentation-level applications that synchronize the user identifier, patient identifier, and/or observation identifier across multiple applications for a "single sign-on, single-patient-look-up user experience."

Claims Attachments

Standard Electronic Attachments are a means of electronically exchanging additional information to augment another healthcare transaction. Examples of transactions that may need such attachments include healthcare claims, prior authorizations, referrals, or public health reporting. The goal of Standard Healthcare Attachments is to make the process of submitting and adjudicating healthcare claims (and other transactions if desired) more efficient by providing structured, standardized electronic data to payers.

Clinical Document Architecture

The CDA Release 2.0 provides an exchange model for clinical documents (such as discharge summaries and progress notes)—and brings the healthcare industry closer to the realization of an electronic medical record. By leveraging the use of XML, the HL7 Reference Information Model (RIM) and coded vocabularies, the CDA makes documents both machine-readable (so they are easily parsed and processed electronically) and human-readable (so they can be easily retrieved and used by the people who need them). CDA documents can be displayed using XML-aware Web browsers or wireless applications such as cell phones. Release 2.0 shares the simplicity of rendering and clear definition of clinical documents formulated in

Release 1.0. It provides state-of-the-art interoperability for machine-readable coded semantics as well. CDA Release 2.0 is based on the HL7 Clinical Statement model, is fully RIM-compliant and capable of driving decision support and other sophisticated applications.

Electronic Health Record/Personal Health Record

The HL7 EHR System Functional Model provides a reference list of functions that may be present in an Electronic Health Record System (EHR-S). The function list is described from a user perspective with the intent to enable consistent expression of system functionality. This EHR-S Model, through the creation of Functional Profiles, enables a standardized description and common understanding of functions sought or available in a given setting (e.g. intensive care, cardiology, office practice in one country or primary care in another country).

Structured Product Labeling

Often know as "product labels", "package inserts", or "prescribing information", these documents contain the authorized published information that accompanies any medicine licensed by a medicines licensing authority. The SPL specification is a document markup standard that specifies the structure and semantics of these documents and is similar to the HL7 Clinical Document Architecture (CDA).

7.5.4 HL7 Standards Referenced by HHS Final Rule

Four HL7 standards are listed in the Final Rule issued by the U.S. Department of Health and Human Services that included an Initial Set of Standards, Implementation Specifications, and Certification Criteria for Electronic Health Record Technology. In this section, we will review these four standards in detail and the purpose for which they have been referenced.

7.5.4.1 Clinical Document Architecture

The Clinical Document Architecture (CDA) Release 2.0 proposes a model for the exchange of clinical documents including discharge summaries and progress notes which are a part of the usual Electronic Medical Records. CDA is based on XML, the HL7 Reference Information Model (RIM) and coded vocabularies.

The documents generated by CDA are both machine readable and human readable. This ensures that they can be processed by computers (aiding automation) and can also be read and used by clinicians to make clinical decisions. Because CDA documents are based on XML format, they can be displayed by any tool or software that display XML format, and specialized readers are not necessary. Many web browsers are capable of displaying XML documents. In addition, there are natively available XML readers on most platforms including PCs and hand-held devices. Similarly, any XML-capable repository can manage CDA. CDA documents are therefore ideally suited for clinical use involving human touch points, as well as sophisticated applications that rely on automation.

CDA specifies the syntax and also provides a framework for specifying the full semantics of any clinical document which is assumed to have the following six characteristics: Persistence, Stewardship, Potential for authentication, Context, Wholeness, Human readability.

A CDA document can contain any type of clinical content. Typical Clinical documents such as Discharge Summaries, Imaging Reports, Admission & Physical reports, Pathology Reports etc can therefore be generated in the form of CDA documents.

CDA documents can have different levels of Semantic Interoperability. Full semantic interoperability is when a document can be used in any application, even if it wasn't designed for that application. So a document with full semantic interoperability can be created for one purpose, like a public health report or for transfer of care, but can be interpreted by other applications with the same degree of confidence that a human would use the information. The "level" of a CDA document refers to the degree to which a receiver can expect to drive automated processes. A Level One CDA has no requirements beyond the standard header metadata and human-readability for the body. The header contains a number of XML-encoded metadata fields (such as provider name, document type, document identifier, and so on) which allow it to be filed, searched, categorized and retrieved. The body itself is not encoded, but contains data in commonly used formats such as PDF or .DOC, or a .JPG (image file). This means it is readable at the point of care by a physician. A Level Two CDA specifies a coded header as in Level One, with the body of the document compliant with the XML format with sections and sub-sections that are coded. A Level Three CDA contains the same expectations as Levels One and Two, plus it contains coded information within the sections including the full specification of the HL7 Reference Information Model (RIM) and controlled vocabulary such as LOINC, SNOMED, ICD, CPT and so on.

XML tags by themselves cannot support clinical system interoperability. The XML tags in a CDA document are defined by the HL7 Reference Information Model (RIM) which is based on a variant of Unified Modeling Language (UML) and has been developed by literally hundreds of thousands of hours of collaborative work by practitioners, scientists, vendors and implementers over a decade. The CDA specification details the relationship of the documents to the model and contains a refined model (RMIM) which takes RIM classes and further constrains them to define the precise parameters of a clinical document.

CDA documents are already in widespread use worldwide for exchanging healthcare-related information. In the US, Regional Health Information Organizations (RHIOs) as well as Military Health Organizations intend to use CDA formats, and therefore anyone who needs to communicate with RHIOs needs to be capable of generating CDA documents. Academic Medical Centers and Research Institutions are also implementing CDA. Examples are the Mayo Clinic, Columbia-Presbyterian in New York, Duke Clinical Research Institute, etc. Many commercially available Healthcare IT systems already generate documents that are CDA-compliant. This includes vendors of EHR systems, Practice Management systems, dictation/transcription systems, etc. Examples of CDA messages are provided in an appendix.

7.5.4.2 Continuity of Care Document (CCD)

The Continuity of Care Document (CCD) specifies the structure, coding and semantics of a patient summary clinical document. CCD was developed as a collaborative effort combining ASTMs Continuity of Care Record (CCR) and the HL7 Clinical Document Architecture (CDA) specifications with the objective of creating a single consolidated standard for healthcare documents. Prior to the CCD, users either adopted the CDA standard or the CCR standard— both of which are intended for the same purpose. However, users of

CDA standard could not communicate with users of CCR standard and vice versa. By consolidating the two into a common format, it was hoped that the use of Electronic Health Records and Electronic Communication of medical data would become more prevalent thereby leading to better patient care, safety, quality and efficiency. Further, it was hoped that the consolidated standard would be widely compatible with existing systems already in use.

[Note: Like the CDA discussed in the earlier section, the CCR is also an XML-based standard used for clinical data exchange, i.e., to aid the transition of a patient from one healthcare provider to another. It was developed by ASTM International, and unlike a comprehensive EHR, the CCR only provides a snapshot of treatment and basic patient information. This includes the diagnosis and reason for referral rather than the symptoms and treatment chronology from one or more visits]

Further support for this consolidated standard was provided by CCHIT which made it a part of their certification criterion for EHR products. CCHIT criteria for emergency department EHR products/vendors require all ambulatory and inpatient EHRs to be CCD compatible—meaning they should be able to send and receive clinical documents in the CCD format. Most vendors will therefore implement CCD in their EMR systems, and consequently most care providers will begin using it as well.

CCD has been designed to support the import, export and management of XML data which is typically required from a typical EMR. Although it is based on CDA elements, the data itself is defined by CCR. This is done by defining a set of templates for the CDA elements. Within each template, the scope of the clinical data is as per CCR. Templates can have supporting templates if required. The templates defined within CCD are:

1) Header
2) Purpose
3) Problems
4) Procedures
5) Family history
6) Social history
7) Payers

8) Advance directives

9) Alerts

10) Medications

11) Immunizations

12) Medical equipment

13) Vital signs

14) Functional stats

15) Results

16) Encounters

17) Plan of care.

The purpose of the CCD specification is to allow the exchange of clinical data, and make it available at the point of care. It allows providers to share clinical summary information about patients to referring physicians, pharmacies, with EMR systems and other providers. This summary information is provided in the overall context of the patient's EHR. The summary contains the relevant administrative, demographic, and clinical information facts about a patient's healthcare. It covers one or more healthcare encounters of the patient. Any healthcare provider (either a practitioner or an automated system) is in a position to aggregate the pertinent data about a patient and forward it to another healthcare provider. The CCD can also include free flow text (unstructured text) along with standardized information. This allows the receiving physician to view this text narrative while providing continued care.

The advantage of all of this for the patient is that integrity of data is maintained (data is not lost or modified) when it is transferred from one practitioner to another.

For example, an EMR system in a pathological lab can print out a CCD document based on a patient's test result. This CCD document can either be forward to the healthcare provider (which initiated the test) or can also be printed out for the benefit of the patient.

As per AHIMA/CAST, The following are examples of scenarios where CCD can be used for communicating healthcare information:

1) Sending Summary of Care or other clinical information from a Nursing Home/Clinic/PT/OT/CCRCto Personal Health Record system

2) A older patient's Family providing the patient's Health Summary to Adult Day Care Center

3) Health Records maintained by Individuals over their lifespan

4) Sending patient Records from one provider (nursing home/ hospital/clinic/acute care center/Emergency) to another.

5) Exchanging health records between Home care/Assisted Living/ Nursing Homes

6) Attending physician to nursing homes

7) Maintaining and exchanging records over the duration of management Cancer treatment, Chronic Care Management, Nutrition Consultation

8) For administrative documents such as Managed Care Pre-Certification Request, Part D Pre-Certification, Billing Attachments, Nursing Home Data Reporting, Home Care Data Reporting

9) For research-related applications

10) For HIPAA Claims Attachment Rule

Examples of CCD messages are provided in an appendix.

7.5.4.3 Messaging Standard Version 2.3.1 and 2.5.1

HL7's Version 2.x messaging standard is the most widely implemented standard for healthcare in the world. It supports not only clinical processes, but also administrative, and financial processes. It allows interoperability between the various IT systems in a practice such as practice Management systems, patient admission systems, pharmacy and billing systems and EMR systems. It covers messages for information exchange in the following areas:

- Patient Demographics
- Patient Charges and Accounting
- Patient Insurance and Guarantor
- Clinical Observations
- Encounters including Registration, Admission, Discharge and Transfer
- Orders for Clinical Service (Tests, Procedures, Pharmacy, Dietary and Supplies)

- Observation Reporting including Test Results
- The synchronization of Master Files between systems
- Medical Records Document Management
- Scheduling of Patient Appointments and Resources
- Patient Referrals—Specifically messages for primary care referral
- Patient Care and problem-oriented records.

HL7 v2.x messages are composed of delimited text. They do not use XML. A message consists of data fields which are separated by special termination characters. The data fields need not have a fixed length. For each field, there are rules governing how data is coded within them. Several data fields together form a segment. Like data fields, segments can also be of variable length and two segments are separated by termination characters. At the beginning of each segment is a three-character code that identifies it within the overall message. To locate a specific data field, one locates the segment within which the data field lies and then locates the data field within that segment. Within each data field are components, and each component in turn has several subcomponents. This gives rise to the following hierarchy within a message:

1) Message
2) Segment
3) Fields
4) Components
5) Subcomponents

Examples of Segments within a message include:

1) The Message Header Segment (MSH) which is present in all HL7 messages and defines the HL7 version used, message type, the sender/receiver information and also the formatting information such as the field separators used, the encoding characters, etc.
2) The Patient Identification Segment (PID) which includes all information that identifies the patient, including demographic information.

3) The Financial Transaction Segment (FT1) which includes all the financial information such as the insurance information, billing and payment information, etc.

4) The Observation Reporting Segment (OBR) which actually delineates the start of the report and includes the observation set and related ordering information. This implies one or more OBR segments. Within each OBR segment, some of the data fields pertain to the ordering message and some to the reporting message.

5) The Observation Results Segment (OBX) which is used to transmit a single observation.

7.6 INTEROPERABILITY AND CLOUD-BASED SYSTEMS

HIEs are conceptually a 'Cloud-based service' as far as providers are concerned. HIE infrastructure is hosted on servers in a Datacentre, and is accessible online for the providers to exchange information. Information is exchanged using standard protocols such as HL7. A provider (whether it is a hospital, a clinic or a single physician practice) needs to have internet connectivity if the provider is to access the HIE—either for sending information or receiving information. If a practice does not have an internet connection— i.e., only has an in-house IT infrastructure without the external connectivity, the practice cannot be a part of HIE infrastructure and cannot benefit from it.

From an interoperability perspective, there is an advantage to using Cloud-based systems. Cloud vendors typically are in a better position to ensure high availability i.e., ensuring that systems are 'always ON', and therefore in a position to communicate with other Cloud-based infrastructure such as HIEs. If your IT system needs to communicate with a Cloud-based service, it is advantageous if your system is Cloud-based as well.

Secondly, Interoperability protocols are constantly evolving. Each time a new protocol is added or an existing protocol is modified, an in-house system has to be upgraded to ensure compliance with the modified standard. A Cloud-based system has to be upgraded too, but that is done by the Cloud provider in a manner transparent to the end-user. The end-user does not need to worry either about the communication protocols or when or how the Cloud-based system is upgraded.

The provisioning the bandwidth for data exchange necessary for ensuring interoperability is the responsibility of your Cloud provider rather than you. This can be particularly relevant if you are transferring a large number of images or scans between your system and the HIE.

To summarize, in order to avail the benefits of Interoperability and partner with HIEs, a healthcare IT system needs to have always-on connectivity with HIEs. Secondly, practitioners need to keep upgrading their IT systems each time a new Interoperability standard is introduced. From the perspective of interoperability, it is advantageous for practitioners to use Cloud-based IT systems themselves.

While signing up with a Cloud-based provider, practitioners need to ask if the systems comply with Interoperability requirements.

REFERENCES

[1] Coming to Terms: Scoping Interoperability for Health Care, Health Level Seven, February 2007.

[2] *Principles of Health Interoperability HL7 and SNOMED*, Tim Benson, Springer-Verlag, 2010.

[3] Evolution of State Health Information Exchange/A Study of Vision, Strategy, and Progress, The Agency for Healthcare Research and Quality (AHRQ), Department of Health and Human Services.

[4] http://www.hl7.org

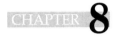

CHAPTER 8

Cloud-based Personal Health Records (PHR)

Personal Health Record (PHR) systems are a set of electronic tools that allow people to access and manage their lifelong health information and make appropriate parts of it available to those who need it [1]. Unlike Clinical EMR systems (in which a patient's medical history is maintained by care providers), in a PHR system, the data is entered, edited, forwarded to others by each individual for himself/herself. Also note that PHR is different from the Patient Portals, which allow the patient to view the information contained in an EMR system of a healthcare provider.

PHR, when diligently maintained, contain a chronological record of every aspect of a person's health related information, including hospitalizations, surgeries & procedures, lab tests and reports, allergies, and even life-style related information.

[*Note: This chapter is addressed to users of PHR. In this chapter, 'you' refers to the patient, and not the provider.*]

The two primary reasons for maintaining a PHR are coordination of care and safety [2]. Over the years, people are likely to obtain healthcare from multiple entities, and meet with different physicians depending on the nature of their requirement at each time. It is also possible that patients are seeing more than one physician simultaneously in relation to more than one complaint. This makes it necessary to consolidate the health care administered by various care providers. The single reason for maintaining a PHR is to have access to your own medical history at any point in time.

PHR systems normally provide ability to store every single piece of information relevant to your health. This information can come from different sources. A typical PHR system contains information such as:

1. Records obtained from a healthcare provider such as records of physical examinations, discharge summaries for hospitalization, surgeries or other procedures
2. Reports of laboratory tests and radiology reports, preventive regimens such as colonoscopies, mammograms, etc.
3. Information about vaccinations
4. Prescriptions
5. Information obtained from insurance provider
6. Information known to and entered by the patient such as family history, allergies/adverse drug reactions, general observations about daily habits and so on.
7. Information tracked by the individual such as weight, cholesterol level, blood pressure, medication effectiveness, and similar data over a period of time
8. Contact information about care providers, insurance company, employer, etc.

Most effective modern PHR systems are Cloud-based. The purpose of maintaining a PHR is to be able to make selective portions of that information available to designated entities at any time at short notice. This means that the PHR has to be stored where it is globally accessible, 24x7. The Cloud is therefore the ideal place to store PHR. Most modern PHR systems have advanced features that make it easy for a person to manage all their health records online using a simple web-browser.

Cloud-based PHR systems have the following capabilities:

1. They allow a person to directly import their data from other healthcare IT systems (supporting compatible formats), such as the EMR systems of their care provider. This makes it easy for the person to keep his/her PHR up to date.

2. They allow a person to define levels of information access thereby providing excellent control in terms of what information is to be made visible to whom.

3. They allow storage of images, scans, etc.

4. They often contain knowledge-bases that provide alerts on adverse drug-drug reactions or drug-allergy information

5. They contain search engines and ability to quickly access informational literature pertaining to your specific conditions.

6. They allow export of all or specific information into standard formats that can be read by other healthcare IT systems if required.

The following are some of the specific benefits resulting from using a PHR system:

1. Maintaining Personal Health Records offer a systematic way to track ones health, providing a single repository for storing all your healthcare related information. Over a period of time a PHR becomes a valuable knowledgebase regarding your own health—including history of your illnesses, treatments prescribed and so on. Maintaining copies of paper-based charts or reports from disparate sources is not easy. Many PHR systems allow you to store digitized/scanned copies of paper-based records. A Cloud-based PHR is not affected by fire, theft or other natural calamities that can destroy paper-based records.

2. Having your PHR available can be invaluable when you do not have access to your regular physician, or when you want to meet a doctor who does not have access to the EMR from your healthcare provider. In such a situation, you can share your PHR with the doctor you are seeing, thereby giving the doctor detailed information about your medical background, and helping understand your problem. If you visit multiple physicians for different reasons, you can consolidate your records from these physicians into your PHR, and provide each of your physicians access to those consolidated records. The PHR is useful if you need to get a second opinion from a consultant or a specialist. Many times, having a PHR also

makes it a lot easier to fill out forms when you visit the doctor—there is no need for clipboards. It is important to note however, that a physician may not necessarily trust information in a PHR, or may not make decisions based purely on information contained therein. Nevertheless, it is useful for a physician to see a documented record of your health than relying on your memory at that moment.

3. Most PHR systems allow you the ability to research educational information online, specifically pertaining to your condition and treatment you have received. You can also access blogs that narrate the experiences of other patients who have experienced similar conditions. Further, there is information on dietary suggestions, nutritional supplements, as well as the state-of-art research being conducted in that particular area of medicine and so on. Having this entire information means that you can ask your doctor the right questions when you go for your appointment. Sometimes, PHRs can also help you cut down on lab tests—if your doctor sees the results of a previous tests, it is possible that you won't have to take them again.

4. Many PHR systems are also linked directly to pharmacies. This allows you to maintain a record of all the drugs or medications you are taking. PHR systems also alert you to possible drug allergies or drug-drug reactions. You can import your prescriptions into your PHR. If you buy your medications from multiple pharmacies, the PHR provides a means to consolidate all prescriptions into a single repository. Some PHRs also allow you to order refills from pharmacies online. PHRs can alert you when you need refills or about physician appointments.

5. Some Cloud-based PHRs support remote monitoring applications by directly integrating with monitoring devices, for example, blood pressure monitors, glucometers, and so on. The readings can be monitored by the provider remotely.

6. Some Cloud-based PHRs allow you to interact with physicians or Nurse practitioners online—either via messenger tools or even via web-conferencing. You can share the data in your PHR during the course of such 'e-visits'.

7. You can store critical information in your PHR such as the contact information of your healthcare providers, physicians, insurance companies, etc which can be useful when you need such information in emergencies.

A study of the benefits of PHR has been made in [1]. The data in that report shows that the maximum benefit of PHR results from third-party PHRs, and in the areas of remote conferencing with physicians, remote monitoring and sharing of prior test results. On the other hand, there are certain aspects one needs to be careful about when using a PHR system.

1) As with all Cloud-based systems, in a PHR system, your data is protected with a password. Anyone who obtains your password can access all your medical information. When it comes to PHR systems, it is a good idea to anonymize all your information before storing it in a PHR system. Anonymization refers to removing all information that can identify you as the owner of that information. For example, this means removing information such as name, contact information, and any other demographic information from your PHR. Many people use an alias instead of a real name for their PHR accounts.

2) The fact that you have a documented medical history can sometimes work against you in case of a dispute with your insurance provider. This is particularly true if you have entered information in your PHR that was not obtained from a healthcare provider.

PHR systems are not required to be HIPAA compliant. When using a PHR, persons should be aware that they are using a system that does not offer the HIPAA safeguards. One therefore relies on an element of trust in the PHR vendor when storing one's health information in the PHR. This trust does not only pertain to ethics of the vendor, but also to the vendor's technical capability to keep your information secure. All PHR systems have their own terms of use and privacy policies. These privacy policies are often written in a way that makes them hard to understand for anyone who is not a lawyer. At the same time, it is necessary to review the privacy policies of the vendor before subscribing to a particular PHR. Specifically, it is important to have clarity on the ownership of the data, who has access to your records, whether the PHR vendor can share your records with a third party, and so on. In certain situations, the PHR vendor's privacy policy may not extend to partners of the vendor that have access to PHR information. In such a situation, one needs to be careful not to expose PHR information to such partners. In [3] is a study that reviews the privacy policies of some of the PHR vendors and grades them as well.

There are several Cloud-based PHR systems available. These are typically backed by three types of entities: insurance companies, healthcare providers and third party vendors. The study in [3] indicates that the PHR systems backed by third party vendors are the most popular. This is probably because individuals typically do not want to volunteer health data to insurance companies, and also want the flexibility of being able to change their health care provider at any time.

We now cover two of the popular third-party backed PHR offerings: Google Health and Microsoft HealthVault.

8.1 GOOGLE HEALTH

Google Health is a Cloud-based personal health record (PHR) system from Google. It has been available since 2008, and at this time is free for individual use. Users can create their PHR accounts and enter their health information online. Google Health also partners with many healthcare providers and pharmacies, and users can automatically import their health information from several healthcare providers into Google Health account. If the user has accessed services at two different healthcare providers the user can actually merge the records into his/her Google Health account. Users have to explicitly permit the access of such information from each healthcare provider; Google does not do so on its own for privacy reasons.

In addition to being able to retrieve, merge and consolidate healthcare records and also enter health information on one's own, Google Health also allows the user to search for Doctors and Hospitals in a particular area, and find health care related information and resources.

The typical user workflow in Google Health involves the following steps:

8.1.1 Creating an account

Users can create a Google Health account either by creating a fresh account on http://www.googlehealth.com or by using their existing Gmail accounts & passwords to login to Google Health directly.

8.1.2 Creating a profile

Creating a profile involves adding basic information to the user account. You can add the following information to your profile:

1) Basic information such as Age, Sex, Height, Weight and so on.
2) Your previously known conditions (select none or more from a alphabetically arranged list of several hundred different conditions).
3) Your present medications. Again, you can select from a list of medications on the site. The list is fairly exhaustive, and covers most common medications.
4) Your known allergies. To be selected from a list of allergies.
5) The nature of surgeries or procedures you have undergone.
6) The medical/laboratory or other tests performed and their results.
7) Your immunization record, which is the summary of immunizations you have received.

8.1.3 Importing Medical Records

Google has partnered with a number of health services organizations such as hospitals, and pharmacies. Also on the partner list are EMR vendors. If you have obtained medical care at one or more of the partner organizations, you can directly import your records from those organizations into your Google Health account. In case your physician or family doctor uses an EMR system from one of the listed software partners, you can import those records into your Google Health account too. The partnerships are not endorsements of either party by the other. They just allow a common user of both systems to authorize movement of data from one system to another.

8.1.4 Health Services

Users of Google Health can avail of several services. These services are offered by Google partners, and are paid services. There are several different types of services, including those for

1) Assessing personal health based on Google Health records,
2) Directly consulting with physicians for problem-specific consultations or second opinions
3) Comparing prescribed medications in terms of effectiveness and cost with other available options
4) Ordering lab tests online
5) Converting old paper-charts to electronic form, and including them as a part of Google Health account.
6) Access to numerous third party applications based on your data in Google Health. You have to subscribe to these applications and explicitly provide permission for them to use your data.
7) Copying your records to a local storage such as a USB drive or sharing them electronically.

8.1.5 Google Health API

Google has also published an API (Application Programming Interface) which allows third parties to develop software and offer it to users of Google Health. This has created a library of software applications for a variety of tasks that users of Google health can buy and use.

8.2 MICROSOFT HEALTHVAULT

Microsoft HealthVault has been built as an online location where individuals can store all their health and fitness-related information. It has been available to users since 2007. MS HealthVault not only allows individuals to store information, but MS HealthVault also offers a platform for other entities to provide services on this platform. This includes entities such as hospitals and healthcare providers, payees or insurance companies, pharmacies, laboratories, employers, healthcare associations, device manufacturers, application developers and so on. We will discuss below how each of these entities can use MS HealthVault.

8.2.1 Individuals

Patients can use a HealthVault record to track their medications, allergies, lab results and other data, using Web applications and personal health and fitness devices. While MS HealthVault is for individuals to maintain their health related information, it is assumed that individuals will only occasionally type in or enter their data into the portal. More frequently, it would be the healthcare providers, pharmacies or other entities permitted by the individual that would feed data into the individual's HealthVault account.

8.2.2 Healthcare Providers

Patients use a HealthVault account to maintain their medical history. Physicians who use compatible IT systems can directly access the patient's data and view the medical history of the patient (The patient actually needs to authorize which information from the HealthVault can be seen by the Physician). This not only saves the patient the effort of having to fill out forms, but the physician is in a better position to evaluate the patient in the context of the patient's medical history and thereby make informed decisions. Patients can also send HealthVault information to participating physicians even if the physician does not have an EMR system.

This applies for hospitals and clinics too. A patient, who walks in seeking care into the hospital for the first time, does not need to fill out forms to share his medical history. It can be done by the patient by sending data from his/her HealthVault account to the clinical IT system of the hospital.

Many devices directly integrate into MS HealthVault, i.e., the readings gathered by the device can be directly imported into a HealthVault account. Physicians can provide improved post-operative care by remotely monitoring the health data that has been imported from devices directly into HealthVault accounts.

Conversely, any information entered by the physician can also be imported directly into their HealthVault by the patient.

8.2.3 Laboratories and Radiology centers

Digitally signed (authenticated) results from Labs and Radiology centers can be directly sent to patient's HealthVault account (assuming such permission is granted by the patient). Lab results obtained on paper or films are hard to retain over a period of time. If they are directly sent to HealthVault, patients can access them at any time thereafter. Furthermore, it saves the patient the effort of having to scan and upload these documents anywhere.

8.2.4 Pharmacies

When Pharmacies are provided access to HealthVault by Patients, pharmacies can monitor medications, prescriptions, etc., and provide services such as mail order fulfillment, and other health monitoring tools.

8.2.5 Device Manufacturers

Device manufacturers can market their devices to a large number of HealthVault users by ensuring that their devices are compatible with MS HealthVault. Microsoft has a set of unified drivers called the HealthVault Connection Center which run on any MS Windows computer. Once these drivers are installed, users can connect any compatible device and upload data from the device directly into the patient's HealthVault accounts. This data then becomes available to other applications that have permissions to access the data. For example, this makes it possible for readings of a glucometer or a BP meter to directly go into the HealthVault account thereby enabling a healthcare provider to monitor them.

8.2.6 Application Developers

The data contained within HealthVault account can be made available to specific applications by the patient. Application Developers in turn can utilize the Microsoft interfaces to write programs that directly allow them to access the HealthVault data of patients who have authorized such an access. There are a large number of applications already available that help patients manage their health, for example for monitoring patients for anxiety or depression, and for automatically calling first responders on basis of warning signs.

8.3 HOME MONITORING

The home monitoring aspect of PHRs is seen by patients and care providers alike as one of its key benefits. As populations age, the number of patients with chronic ailments is growing rapidly, and so is the cost of providing care to them. This is not only an issue for patients and their immediate families but also for governments and tax-payers. According to the Health Council of Canada, almost a third of the population has at least one chronic disease, and those with multiple chronic diseases consume 80% of the public health budget since they are the largest users of healthcare facilities. The Health Council of Canada estimates that over 5.5 million Canadians have chronic diseases which lend themselves to daily monitoring. Utilizing Remote Patient Monitoring (RPM) tools, these patients can reduce the cost per day to the healthcare system from more than $4,000 for acute care to between $30 and $50 for self-care.

The device which monitors vital signs or other specific health parameters is worn or regularly used by the patient. This device collects necessary readings and transmits them to a networking device placed within the patient's home. Devices that transmit information wirelessly are more convenient because they offer the advantage of mobility to the patient. Examples of such monitoring devices are:

1) Glucose meters
2) Weight scales
3) Blood pressure devices
4) Exercise monitoring devices
5) Devices for monitoring insulin levels
6) Devices for detecting vital signs medication and fluid intake
7) Devices for fall detection.
8) Peak flow meters and FEV1 tracking devices
9) Pulse oximeters
10) Pedometers
11) Heart rate monitors

The networking device collects readings from the monitoring device, and further transmits them to a Cloud-based PHR over the internet. The networking device could either be a custom device that directly connects to a networking hub within the household or a device that connects to a PC which in turn transfers information to the Cloud-based PHR over the internet.

The Cloud-based PHR maintains a database of all gathered readings. This information can also be integrated into the provider's EMR system, thereby allowing a physician to view the readings in the context of the patient's overall medical records. PHR systems also have the ability to define rules that trigger an alert to healthcare providers, or other designated entities. Alternately, it is also possible for healthcare providers to view the readings gathered over a period of time.

Based on the nature of the alert received from the PHR, the healthcare provider takes appropriate action, such as either sending emergency help, or prescribing a changed medication, etc. This is shown in Fig. 8.1.

Patient Monitoring via PHR enhances the participation of the patient in the process of delivering care. It allows them to be cared for at home, even if they are based at a location that is geographically remote from the care provider.

Technology solutions that provide the ability to remotely monitor patients with chronic illnesses are an emerging business opportunity for device manufacturers as well as PHR solution providers. According to a report from Parks Associates' [4] the remote health monitoring and disease management industry (including the market for devices and personal health records (PHR)) is likely to be a $460 million industry by 2013.

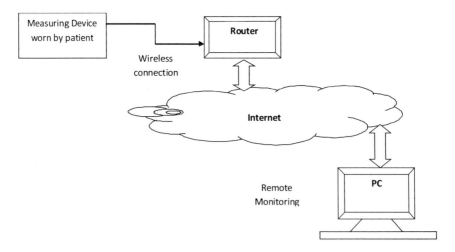

Fig. 8.1 Remote monitoring via a PHR.

8.4 WEB-MEETINGS FOR HEALTHCARE OR EVISITS

An 'eVisit' is a patient-provider encounter that happens electronically, over the Internet. Rather than visit the healthcare provider in person, patients are able to consult their physicians over an electronic medium, from the comfort of their homes. eVisits can be of the following nature:

1) Patients can send messages or emails to their physicians and the physician can respond to the query in the context of the patient's medical records to which the physician already has access.

2) Patients can initiate real-time, live web-based video-conferencing with their healthcare providers, while simultaneously sharing their medical records.

These electronic communications are secure, i.e., they are encrypted and the privacy of the discussion is thereby maintained. Several PHR systems have already integrated such eVisit capability as a part of the overall functionality. Some PHR systems have integrated video conferencing features that allow patients to seek out and talk to a healthcare provider live, at any time with the click of a button on their computer screens.

eVisits are suited for the following situations:

1. Medical situations that are not of an emergent or urgent nature

2. Situations where patients seek follow-up consultation

3. Situations involving chronic ailments

4. Situations where patient requires urgent advice, and is unable to reach the physician personally.

From the perspective of the patient, eVisits provide an additional means of connecting with their physicians at any time, and from the comfort of their homes. It also means avoiding travel to the clinic or spending time in waiting rooms. Normally, the patient-physician interaction during an eVisit is electronically recorded and stored, which means the patient has the ability to revisit the information subsequently if required. This is particularly useful for patients who live far away or do not have access to reliable transportation.

From the perspective of the physicians, the ability of the patient to eVisit certainly provides the physician the ability to provide better continued care. If the physician feels a personal visit is necessary, the physician can always instruct the patient to do so. However, the speed of adopting eVisit capability has been low among physicians. This is because of several reasons. Firstly, physicians feel that they would be overwhelmed with electronic communication from patients and would not have the time to respond to such communication. Secondly, because HIPAA, physicians are apprehensive about the security and privacy issues pertaining to eVisits (and their subsequent liability). Thirdly, because physicians can charge more for personal visits in comparison to eVisits, eVisits are potentially viewed as a loss of revenue.

In [5] the author has considered all of these issues while making the point that eVisits actually aid physicians. eVisits are simply a way of enhancing patient care and saving time for all parties involved. Several health plans nationally are rolling out e-visits including Aetna, Cigna and WellPoint. The typical cost for an e-visit is $30–$50.

The potential for leveraging Cloud-based healthcare and eVisit solutions is enormous. On the one hand, more than 200 million Americans have access to the Internet. More than 60% of patients feel that ability to communicate using email with their doctors would be a positive thing, and that they forget to ask something or other during their appointment with a doctor. About three-quarters of all respondents said they would like to use e-mail to make appointments, receive reminders for visits, and communicate directly with their doctors. More than 30% of patients feel that they are frustrated about not being able to get through to someone who can answer their healthcare related questions or having to provide same information over and over again each time they visit a doctor.

The ability to communicate electronically with physicians would address several of these frustrations, and certainly lead to greater patient satisfaction.

For details of statistics referred to above, kindly refer [6] and [7].

8.5 MOBILE PHR APPLICATIONS

Most mobile devices come with internet browsers, so any Cloud-based application that is browser-accessible is also accessible from a mobile device. This means that any Cloud-based PHR application that can be launched from within a browser is also accessible via a mobile or handheld device.

There are a few reasons however, to think of a mobile device as more than just "yet another device with a browser".

1) Mobile devices are carried on person all the time. This makes them the best device to store a person's medical information that is most likely to be required in case of an emergency.

2) Wireless coverage has blind-spots, i.e., areas where mobile devices cannot access the Internet. Hence, if mobile devices are to be used to access key medical information, that information needs to be stored on the mobile itself rather than being accessible remotely via a browser.

3) Mobile devices have a display screen that is of an entirely different size from the screen of a typical computer. Hence information rendered on a mobile device screen needs to be formatted in order to make it appropriate for viewing on a mobile device.

The best way to address the above points is to develop custom applications for specific mobile platforms. These applications are designed for viewing on a mobile display, and the functionality is organized in a manner that makes it easy to use with the limited keyboard capability of a typical mobile. These applications are not launched from within a browser, but they do access Cloud-based data repositories to access data required for their functionality. In addition, these applications also cache certain key information on the mobile device itself, so that it is accessible even without an active internet connection.

There are numerous mobile-based applications in healthcare. A comprehensive listing of these is available in [8].

Mobile healthcare applications for patients can be broadly divided into four categories:

1) Applications which interface with medical devices (either wearable or implanted) and help monitor their readings. For example, this includes applications where mobile phones directly communicate with devices for monitoring blood pressure, heart rate, blood glucose, etc. The readings are either communicated to a PHR system by the mobile phone, or the mobile application itself analyzes the readings and sends alerts to care providers in case the readings are not satisfactory. There are applications that enable contact with a medical expert if there is a danger of the patient having a cardiac arrest. The mobile phone includes a sensor that measures heart rate and transmits data to a call centre. If the data show the patient is in danger the call centre operator arranges for emergency services to attend the patient. Other applications in this category include those for breath analysis, voice pattern analysis, temperature measurement, weight measurement, sleep monitoring, pulse oximetry, and so on.

2) Applications that help patients access their PHR records. This can be done either via a browser (which is available on most mobile phones), or via specific applications ('native applications') that are resident on the mobile phones, and access and display the PHR information from the Cloud. These 'native applications' are typically easier to use and navigate since they have been written keeping the mobile phone in mind.

3) Applications that store key medical information or identification information so that it is handy in case of emergencies. In these applications, the mobile phone or the SIM card inside it functions as an Identification card or 'Information token'. Mobile phones have adequate storage capacity to store the basic medical information about the owner. They can also store passwords that can be used access the online PHR of a patient in case of emergency. Another example of an interesting application in this category is for patient consent. Details of the surgery such as date, relevant patient information, surgeon's name etc are stored on the mobile phone during a preoperative visit. This information is then verified on the day of the surgery to ensure it is correct.

4) Applications that allow healthcare providers to reach the patient at any time for better delivery of healthcare. In this category of applications, the care provider reaches the patient on his/her mobile phone to communicate time sensitive instructions or other critical health information. Healthcare providers send SMS to their patients reminding them of clinical appointments, time of medication, pharmacy refills, etc. Failure to complete courses of medication, taking incorrect doses, missing a dose, etc are common problems for many patients. SMSs provide time-critical reminders substantially reducing the instances of such problems. Patient Paging (on the patient's mobile) has also been used to enhance the quality of outpatient care. Solutions based on SMS or Paging are relatively simpler to implement and adopt and therefore are very effective.

8.6 GETTING STARTED WITH A PHR

There are many dozens of PHR applications, and it can be difficult to decide which PHR to choose from among the choices available. Sometimes, this is not a matter of personal preference. Your primary healthcare provider or your insurance company may recommend a PHR for you to use.

Assuming the choice of a PHR vendor is your own, the first step is to identify the type of PHR that is appropriate for you. The Amercian Heart Association has created a simple quiz, which you should take in order to determine the PHR system that is most appropriate for you [9]. The choices are between storing your records on your home PC, or storing them online in a system accessible over the internet, or storing them in portable storage devices such as USB drives, or simply storing paper-based records. Depending upon your comfort using the technology and the level of comfort sharing health information, the result of the quiz recommends a system that is best suited for you.

If you arrive at the conclusion that an online (Cloud-based) system is the most appropriate for you, the following additional issues should be thought through before concluding which system is the most suitable for your needs:

1) Type of Vendor. The first thing to decide is the nature of the vendor you want to work with. There are three types of PHR

systems—Those provided by healthcare providers, those provided by insurance companies and third-party promoted systems. If your primary healthcare provider recommends a particular PHR system or your insurance company does that, you may want to consider those systems and their benefits. Nothing however, prevents any individual from using one of the many third-party systems available to the public.

2) Determine the nature of your need. If you need a PHR for monitoring chronic illnesses or want anytime access to your provider or have a condition that makes it necessary to reach a physician at any time, you may want to consider a PHR supported by your provider. Nature of the need also pertains to how you want to use the PHR—whether you want to monitor your own health or want to monitor and manage all health related information about your family.

3) A list of PHRs is available here [10]. It is very important to read and understand the privacy and security policies of the vendor before committing your data to the system. Most vendors publish a privacy policy upfront. It is important read the privacy policy and understand under what circumstances (if any) the vendor can make your data available to a third party.

4) The next stage is to evaluate the functionality you need in the PHR system. You need to be able to store all information that impacts your health into the PHR system. This includes at a minimum:

   a. Your Personal Identification, including name, birth date, and Social Security number. You may decide to not store this information, and rather use an alias.

   b. Emergency contacts such as names and addresses of healthcare providers, physicians, specialists, immediate relatives, etc.

   c. Health insurance information

   d. A chronological record of your medical encounters including illnesses, hospitalizations, surgeries and procedures, along with discharge notes.

  e. Prescriptions, Medications along with dosages
  f. Immunization record
  g. Information about Allergies and hereditary conditions
  h. Lab and radiology results, scans, eye and dental records
  i. Permission forms for release of information
  j. Advance directives, will, etc.

  If you are interested in monitoring the readings from a device you wear, make sure that device is supported by the PHR system. If you will primarily access the PHR from a mobile phone, ensure it is possible to do so. Additionally it is useful if the PHR system allows you to store images and scans of prior records. Finally, it should be easy to import data into the system in standard electronic formats, and the system should also provide you with the ability to only share very specific information from the PHR with anyone you designate. Not only can you determine the supported functionality from the documentation provided, but many PHR systems also provide you the ability to open and test a free trial account.

5) Some PHRs are free, and some are supported by targeted advertisements. While free systems are attractive, it is important to ensure that the vendor is a stable entity likely to be in business for many years.

An excellent resource that helps you in the process of selecting a PHR is [11]. Another resource is here [12]. Several useful forms are available from [13].

Once a PHR system is selected, you need to ask your healthcare providers for all your medical records in an electronic format and import them into your PHR system. Several other pieces of required information in a PHR have to be filled manually by you. You must familiarize yourself with how you can refill prescriptions from your PHR, and how you can share only portions of information from your PHR with others. It is also important to keep the PHR updated on a regular basis.

If you are a physician, or a care provider, it is a good idea to evaluate the available PHR systems and recommend one of these to your patients.

REFERENCES

[1] http://www.ncbi.nlm.nih.gov/pmc/articles/PMC2655982/

[2] http://www.fortherecordmag.com/archives/030310p14.shtml

[3] http://patientprivacyrights.org/personal-health-records/

[4] http://www.researchandmarkets.com/research/72d2bb/disease_management

[5] http://www.transformed.com/e-Visits/e-Visits_There_Yet.cfm

[6] http://www.harrisinteractive.com/news/index.asp?NewsID=166&HI

[7] http://www.illuminas-global.com/images/blog/illumninas_one_in_three_americans_report_re_health_care_pr.pdf

[8] http://www.themobilehealthcrowd.com/?q=node/8

[9] http://www.americanheart.org/downloadable/heart/flash/phrquiz/quiz.html

[10] http://www.open.medicdrive.org/index.php/List_of_PHR_vendors_in_market_today

[11] http://library.ahima.org/xpedio/groups/public/documents/ahima/bok1_032260.hcsp?dDocName=bok1_032260

[12] http://www.myphr.com/index.php/start_a_phr/choose_a_phr/

[13] http://www.pamf.org/healtheducation/medical/phr.html

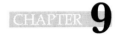

CHAPTER 9

Case Studies

Healthcare practices that are considering the adoption of web-based solutions are likely to benefit from experiences of other practices that have adopted such solutions. In this chapter, we bring two case studies from vendors of web-based solutions for small practices.

[Note: These studies have been contributed by the respective vendors and have been included as submitted. Their inclusion does not indicate an endorsement of the content or the particular solutions.]

9.1 WAITING ROOM SOLUTIONS CASE STUDY

Waiting Room Solutions Inc. is a provider of Cloud-based solutions to various specialties of clinical practices. The following case study demonstrates the adoption of their services by a specific healthcare practice.

This case-study was provided by Nora Alexander, Waiting Room Solutions Inc. with Steven J. Dubin, MD, Ear Nose and Throat of Syracuse.

9.1.1 About the System—Waiting Room Solutions

Waiting Room Solutions (WRS) is a web native, end-to-end, enterprise level solution. It is a web-based application that features an integrated patient portal website, patient registration, scheduling, practice administration, electronic health records, and revenue cycle management. At its heart is a robust EMR that incorporates customizable, specialty-specific content and connectivity to outside entities such as labs, pharmacies, and other medical offices.

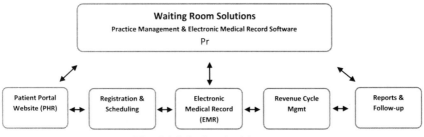

Fig. 9.1 Solution Architecture.

9.1.2 About the Practice — Ear Note and Throat of Syracuse

Ear Nose and Throat of Syracuse is a leading Otolaryngology practice serving patients of all ages in the greater Syracuse, NY Community for over 35 years. They offer full-service Otolaryngology Care including head & neck surgery, audiology, and allergy care. In addition, they offer a unique combination of diagnostic services, including advanced, audio, imbalance, allergy (combined blood and skin), and immunotherapy testing.

The practice has one main location and works in affiliation with four regional hospitals and surgical centers in the greater Syracuse Area. It employs fifteen full-time employees, including two MDs, an Allergy RN, a licensed audiologist and several physician assistants. The highest professional standards have been met in this practice with each physician certified by the American Board of Otolaryngology and Head & Neck Surgery; Audiologists attaining Masters Degree or higher; and physician assistants processing all required certifications. Throughout its long and successful history, the practice has always strived to offer excellence in patient care while sustaining an efficient business model.

9.1.3 Reasons for Selecting a Cloud-based System

Approximately four years ago, Ear Nose and Throat of Syracuse faced issues with the inefficiencies of paper charts, logistics of an outdated and costly practice management system, and escalating expenses. In response, they decided to replace their aging, client-server-based on-site practice management system and move away from paper charting to leverage the benefits of electronic medical records. The practice set out to find a single solution that would address all of their practice management, EMR and billing needs.

Their goal was to eliminate paper charts, enhance patient care, and lower costs; while meeting all federal government regulations and incentives for EMR usage. The practice leadership decided that that an integrated, web-based practice management/EMR system would offer the most comprehensive solution to meet their needs.

Steven Dubin, MD, Lead Provider charged with selection of an EMR, stated "We were generally happy with the previous system. It was easy to use and reliable, but it required daily backups, local server/hardware installation, and update installation. The largest factor in our decision to switch was the need for a complete solution. We wanted to incorporate an EMR into our practice."

The practice had no previous experience with an integrated system. Practice providers were not familiar with electronic charting and only a portion of the staff had experience with the use of the previous server-based scheduling/billing software.

"The selection of a web-based system with a subscription model would help us avoid the needed maintenance and costs of our sever-based systems, while being able to chart a wide variety of patient encounters in a more convenient and professional manner, and make a serious commitment to move our practice technology into the 21st century" Dr. Dubin added.

9.1.4 Practice Product Selection and Vendor Evaluation

The practice created an EMR selection team that included Steven Dubin, MD and Nancy Crast, practice manager (retired). Early in the search process, Dubin and Crast made the decision to move from paper charts to a paperless automate operations, by implementing a web-based practice management and electronic health record (EHR) solution. In this effort they were backed 100% by the efforts and resources of the entire practice staff.

Dr. Dubin stated "Our paper charting was a mess. It was hard to control and clinical information was not organized in an efficient manner. We saw this as an opportunity to address the issues associated with our paper workflow and increase efficiency."

A detailed and careful search led the practice to Waiting Room Solutions. With this selection, the practice leveraged the many benefits of a web-based application within a convenient end-to-end solution. Waiting Room Solutions' Practice Management

System, Version 3, is a CCHIT Certified® 2006 Ambulatory EHR, that provides an integrated suite of solutions designed to support clinical and business workflow that is required to run a medical practice business. It is a web-native application that allows users to access all parts of the system from a standard Internet connection. The result was a selection and implementation process that proved to be an overwhelming success.

Dr. Dubin states "We wanted to have a comprehensive system. Waiting Room Solutions was a comprehensive, end-to-end solution. We chose the system based on the EMR—the specific setup for Otolaryngology and allergy was a large plus."

9.1.5 Minimal IT Requirements

The practice chose to re-outfit their entire IT infrastructure in order to compliment the implementation. It was decided that antiquated computer equipment would be replaced with a state-of-the-art hardware. Time was devoted to select the correct IT vendor for hardware setup and installation. During the IT selection process, the practice learned that the web-based application was far more flexible, and required far less overhead, than their previous in-house system. Waiting Room Solutions' web-based offering required minimal IT expenditure. They were not forced to purchase expensive servers and other centralized equipment.

"We liked the idea that we could control and customize the setup of our computers. We tried to get IT vendors to help us along with that, and in the end there was really only one that would seem to take the time to really hear us out and present us with a coherent proposal. The IT vendor that we went with kind of stood out from the rest" added Dr. Dubin.

As a web-based application, Waiting Room Solutions hardware requirements are straight forward, cost-efficient and flexible. The minimum setup requirements included a basic Internet connection (1.5 mbps download and .75 mbps upload), workstations with a minimum of 1 GB RAM, 2GHz Pentium processor, 17" monitors (dual monitors suggested), laser printer, and document scanner.

Dr. Dubin stated "As far as hardware setup, we mostly followed the lead of the Waiting Room Solutions recommendations. Overall we were as satisfied with how that went, as well as we could have been."

9.1.6 Product Updates

In addition to selecting an appropriate EMR, the practice also wanted to get away from the need to maintain a site-based server and its related equipment. Flexibility and portability of a web-based architecture was priority. They no longer wanted to be subject to performing required, manual updates on an ongoing basis. These updates caused disruption to the practice workflow and mandated the ongoing cost IT services.

Waiting Room Solutions eliminated these issues immediately. All updates were done automatically, without any needed practice work. Updates were performed on weekends exclusively to minimize any potential disruption of patient workflow. The practice was informed in advance to the nature of the anticipated enhancements and updates and release notes were issued.

9.1.7 Cost Savings

From a business perspective, Waiting Room Solutions offered the ability to pay a monthly subscription fee in lieu of the outright fees. This was much more cost effective than the traditional license purchase required by other systems.

"The fact that we did not have to purchase a license, or pay ongoing monthly support fees, was far more effective for the Practice. We were not forced to buy from a specified vendor. Our previous system, for example, had a monthly maintenance cost. We preferred the way Waiting Room Solutions did it. It was far more economical" Dr. Dubin added.

9.1.8 Features—Connectivity and Accessibility

Waiting Room Solutions System offered the practice instant access to patient charts and financial information from any Internet connection. This provided unprecedented convenience in access while enabling internal office communications from any location. Burdensome functions like software updates, security management and backups are all handled centrally. Data corruption, which plagues many client server systems, is managed through proprietary data integrity algorithms and systems. As federal and state security and privacy rules change, the system adapts to insure that that the practice is always compliant.

Waiting Room Solutions has moved Ear, Nose and Throat of Syracuse beyond the traditional 4 walls of their practice... sending, retrieving, filing, and recording information from third parties such as pharmacies, labs, other medical offices and patients is managed for all of these connections and supporting data. The system automatically connected the practice to pharmacies, insurers, labs, other physicians and patients.

"The web-based ability to access the practice from home has been a big benefit. I was coming to the office to do all of my charts on Saturdays. I am now able to chart from my home and other locations... it changed the way I work... the staff has access from home in the case of a snow day... the change was all very positive. I am here at a surgery center today, I am able to do my procedure note and it is automatically going to my biller to generate the claim" Dr. Dubin stated.

The use of Waiting Room Solutions also added a customizable patient website portal for Ear Nose and Throat of Syracuse. It is completely linked to its backend systems. The practice website was easily customized with practice information and patient educational links. This patient portal has provided the practice with a new and higher integrated and efficient communication system with its

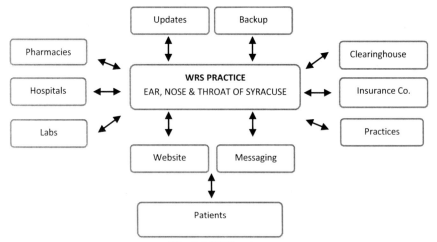

Fig. 9.2 WRS setup.

patients. Patient reminders, notification of test results and general questions can all be transacted seamlessly and securely though the patient portal.

9.1.9 Features—Patient Portal Website with Integrated Registration and Scheduling

The online patient registration offered the practice a convenient, accurate means for patients to provide their critical medical history and patient data. Patients were now able to complete their registration forms from the convenience of their own home—or from anywhere there is an Internet connection. Patients can input their demographic, insurance and health information into a secure, personalized health record. This information would then be accessible to the staff and providers during the office encounter.

Patient's medications, allergies, previous medical history, surgical history, social history, family history and immunization status could be filled out by the patient before they arrived at the practice on the day of the visit. Patients are also able to securely message with the practice through the website. This functionality offered ways to improve practice efficiency with the ability to answer secure messages online, freeing up phone lines and reducing unnecessary fax activity.

9.1.10 Features

Automated Patient Phone Call and Email Reminders

Ear Nose and Throat of Syracuse also took advantage of the completely integrated web based appointment reminder system within the scheduling system. They no longer had to deal with expensive and inaccurate interfaces to external systems. When a patient appointment is made, the system automatically calls and emails that patient with a reminder of the appointment. The system also leveraged VOIP technology so that each call was a fraction of the cost of the standard phone company charges.

Specialty Specific Content for ENT

The solution includes templates and forms that are completely customized for Otolaryngology and Allergy practices, including a Skin Endpoint Titration (SET) Allergy module that automatically calculates end points and vial concentrations; an Audiology Module that allowed the audiologist to chart directly into the system and a fully integrated Scheduling & EMR which integrates with a Billing System that was optimized for ENT charge capture and coding.

> "Waiting Room Solutions has continually been enhanced over the course of the last three years. Most of the updates and added functionality is very helpful and intuitive. For example knowing what tests are due for a patient… that's all a function of being web-based. Everybody else has to wait for a quarterly update… we have any new items instantly."

Customizable EMR

The system offered flexibility and customization to all providers at Ear, Nose and Throat of Syracuse. They were now able to take advantage of specialty-specific content based on their charting preferences. Providers could input data from the keyboard, a tablet, voice recognition, dictation, or handwriting recognition depending on their individual preference.

Dr. Dubin states "One of the strengths of the system in that it was is so broadly adaptable… the ability to do voice recognition, dictation, templates, and the pen, doesn't allow for any excuses for providers not to get on with using Waiting Room Solutions".

Charges were automatically captured, cross checked to payer rules and entered for claim submission without the need for dual entry by the staff. The system's intelligent E&M checker lets the practice staff know the levels of documentation necessary, as the providers were charting.

"The record is now of a much higher quality. It is much easier to know where items are located during the clinical process. Before this system, our paper charting was a mess. This has really streamlined our documentation" Dubin Stated.

ERx (E-Prescribing)

The system brought to the practice benefits of electronic prescribing, with formulary checking through Rx Hub and SureScripts, electronic connections to retail and mail order pharmacies. These functions offered the practice an immediate and accurate transfer of information; saving time and hassles with prescription and refill processing.

"The eRx functionality is fantastic. It saves time and makes the refill process more efficient" Dr. Dubin commented.

It also improved the practice's ability to write and issue prescriptions more accurately and timely with electronic connections to pharmacies. With electronic prescribing and formulary management they saved staff and patient time, while ensuring that prescriptions are accurate and updated. The practice did not need to worry about integration and connectivity with pharmacies.

Integrated Document Management

The system made the practice transition from paper to electronic charts virtually seamless. Its powerful document management solution allowed the practice to scan and index their old paper patient records, so that they could instantly access any paper document from their online practice.

Also included is an Online Fax Service. This offered Ear, Norse and Throat of Syracuse a fully integrated solution in the laboratory management workflow. They could now quickly and easily file electronic faxes directly into patient charts. This saved hours of work each day reviewing charts, laboratory results and radiology results.

Revenue Cycle Management

The Billing module offered the practice functionality for charge collection. Charges are automatically captured, cross checked to payer rules and entered for claim submission without the need for dual entry by the practice staff. The E&M checker let the practice staff know the level of documentation necessary as they charted. All claims were centrally created, scrubbed and submitted.

Autoposting and Eligibility

The solution includes the capability of Autoposting. The practice was now able to view electronic payments and postings in a convenient queue. They could finish the payment entry work in a fraction of the time taken earlier. Further more, the system also includes auto eligibility checking. Prior to the patient's appointment, eligibility was checked to ensure that the practice would be paid for the visit. Clear eligibility messages were displayed to the practice front desk staff to alert them to potential issues with a patient's insurance coverage.

9.1.11 Target Users

Waiting Room Solutions offers Practice Management and EMR solutions to medical practices of all geographic locations, medical specialties and sizes. Target demographic includes 1 to 10 provider's practices. The system is designed for medical doctors, nurse practitioners and physicians assistants of all medical specialty areas. Target users should have basic computer skills and be comfortable using web-based applications. These users should have the capability to participate in remote setup and training activities.

9.1.12 Security and Privacy of the Data

Waiting Room Solutions architecture is designed for virtually unlimited scalability and includes fail-safe data storage (redundancy, mirrored, etc.). It features load balancing, clustered in real time. Daily back up off site and on site is performed on all systems. The solution uses 256 bit encryption and SSL (Secure Sockets Layer) for all data communications, and all internal system communications, between the various layers in the N-tier architecture. SSL (secure sockets) provide security and confidentiality for patient information. The system is hosted in a guarded and locked, secure facility with retinal scan and other biometric authentication. All firewalls and switches are redundant. It meets or exceeds all current HIPAA, State and Federal Privacy and Security requirements.

"Security and Safety has always been at the forefront of Waiting Room Solutions. Our commitment to HIPAA and all Federal, State and local requirements is evidenced by the decisions and outcomes that we have achieved as an EMR and PM system. Our hosting facility provides a level of unsurpassed security and protection. We will continue to lead the way to ensure that our clients and their patients' information is protected and secured at the highest level" said Lawrence Gordon, MD/CEO.

9.1.13 HIPAA and HITECH Compliance

Waiting Room Solutions employs proven, state-of-the-art technology and is able to take advantage of new technologies to meet current and future patient care needs. The system is capable of communicating with other governmental and proprietary systems.

The solution employs state-of the art open source technologies which ensures interoperability and lasting standards. The system is built with Open Source Tools on a LAMP stack of Linux, Apache, MySQL and PHP. It conforms to all standards advocated by the federal government through the National Health Information Infrastructure. The system's messaging standards include: HL7 for clinical data, X12 for financial transactions and EDI, NCPDP for ERx, DICOM for medical images, and IEEE standards for device integration. Data standards include CPT for coding and order identifiers, ICD-9CM and ICD-10CM for diagnosis coding, data mapping to LOINC and SNOMED for clinical terminology and the National Drug Code standards for medication and prescription data.

Waiting Room Solutions meets the requirements of the Medicare PQRI Initiatives, ERx Incentives and the Health Information Technology for Economic and Clinical Health (HITECH) Act, a component of the American Recovery and Reinvestment Act of 2009 (ARRA).

The system subscribes to open source principals and does not use any proprietary (closed) systems or standards within its architecture. This ensures that client practices have interoperability and offers ability to connect to other systems.

9.1.14 Transition Process

"For anyone who takes on transitioning an office from paper to EMR, it's just hard work… no matter what the circumstances might be. Our staff knew that there was no going back. I think that after the exhaustion of the first couple of months, they began to enjoy using it" stated Dr. Dubin.

Any successful implementation of a HIT solution is based on planning, training and practice analysis. In the process of the

ENTS implementation, the Waiting Room Solutions Team collected information about its existing procedures and protocols, performed an analysis, and used the results to guide them through the implementation process.

"The practice developed and put a plan in place for implementation. Regular meetings with the staff were conducted to inform the staff of the vision for implementation. There was really no push back from the staff. Everyone hated the situation of paper charts and the disorganization of the practice prior to this implementation. So, that made it much easier to have everyone buys into the concept of the new system. Everyone fed off of the enthusiasm of the practice leadership. The practice was setting itself up for the future… for the long term. Employees wanted to feel good about the practice" Dubin added.

Waiting Room Solutions in-house support and training staff worked hand-in-hand with their national inventory of Resellers and partners to achieve a successful implemention of their solution. Additionally, they made available a vast library of self guided training videos online.

"We gave the practice manager, unqualified support from the entire practice team. It was a hard process. It is always a challenge moving from paper to EMR. They knew that there was no going back. After that initial first couple of months they saw the benefit and enjoyed using it"stated Nora Alexander, Director of Implementation and Training.

Waiting Room Solutions divides the implementation process into four main leadership areas: Administrative, Clinical Analysis, Network/IT, and Billing. The practice designated leadership roles in each of these crucial areas. Instead of phasing in the use of the system in steps, the practice decided to go-live with the entire system (scheduling, EMR, and billing) at the same time. Patient demographics were imported electronically into the solution. Schedules were loaded in advance by the practice staff. Patient's previous EMR paper charts were scanned and uploaded in preparation for upcoming appointments. Providers worked with both paper and EMR for the beginning of implementation.

Dr. Dubin said "In terms of the transition, the computer part was fairly straight-forward. It was a six month process from start to finish. We deliberately decreased our schedules for the first three months. We did this to build in time to learn and use the new system, removing some of the time pressures of the regular patient workload. We gradually moved to electronic charting over the course of six months. Some providers and staff were early adaptors and charted very quickly, others took longer to embrace the process. Challenges included getting staff to adapt to an electronic system and move away from paper charts. With 15+ people in the office and everyone having an important role, it was imperative that everyone was on board. Even if only two or three of these employees are going to be particularly stressed, or not functioning well with it, then that is a problem for everybody."

"Training was conducted remotely; with Waiting Room Solutions training staff on-site for the first few days of go-live. This was a challenge rather than having an extensive on-site training program."

"For the most part if employees aren't talking about it on a daily basis... it probably means that it is going fine. A lot of update training is done by users sharing knowledge around the office."

9.1.15 Top Benefits of Migrating to a web-based solution

Back in 2007, the leadership of Ear Nose and Throat of Syracuse made the decision to move from paper charts and automate operations by implementing a web-based practice management and electronic health record (EHR) solution. They saw this as an opportunity to address the issues associated with paper workflow and increase efficiencies in their business model. The result was a selection and implementation process that proved to be an overwhelming success.

"Getting rid of charts eliminated at least a half time employee just working on chart management. This was a cost saving measure of itself" Dubin said.

The use of Waiting Room Solutions integrated, web-based system increased practice efficiency and saved money. They were able to do more, with less people.

"Over time were able to consolidate our staff. When we saw an opportunity to consolidate, we did. We found on a couple of occasions that we were able to do more with less people. A large part of it was that we figured out how we could use the system more and not have to depend on replacing somebody that was otherwise leaving. This did not happen until approximately a year into the usage of the solution "added Dr. Dubin.

The monthly subscription model also proved to be an economical benefit to the practice. They no longer had to pay expensive support and maintenance fees that were part of their previous server-based system. A fee based on the number of providers using the application worked in their favor.

"This is a very cost effective solution, as well. We were able to take advantage of paying less when one provider retired and left the practice. The subscription model was a good model and we are glad that we signed on to this model" said Dr. Dubin.

"On the flip side, each provider uses the system differently. Some still opt to use alternative methods of charting (scan into EMR, dictation). That is just the nature of providers. We had to spend a good deal of time, adding extra help, to get the provider to use the system" Dr. Dubin commented.

Over the course of the last three years, the pairing of Ear, Nose and Throat of Syracuse and Waiting Room Solutions' web-based offering proved to be a resounding success. Dr. Dubin looks forward to a bright and exciting future for his practice, as his business and patient care continue to evolve.

"We are very satisfied over the course of a three year experience. During these years there have been incredible changes. The Cloud-based solution from Waiting Room Solutions filled every role to make our process work. Beginning with our initial implementation, everything has been fantastic."

9.2 MITOCHON SYSTEMS CASE STUDY

This case study was provided by Andre Vovan, MD, MBA, Mitochon Systems, Inc.

9.2.1 Background

Mitochon Systems, Inc. a Newport Beach, CA based provider of healthcare solutions has created a HIE/EMR/PHR solution in the cloud to build Virtual Medical Communities and networks of independent physician providers who work together to deliver integrated healthcare services. Mitochon's mission is to transform not just a single physician office, but entire communities of physician offices from their current systems involving use of paper, phone, and faxes as a means of communication to using virtual integrated health delivery systems that rely on secure messaging, electronic medical records, E prescribing, patient portal, and Health Information exchange.

The integrated EMR/HIE/PHR platform called Virtual Medical Community (VMC™) has all capabilities required to meet or exceed "Meaningful Usage" criteria of the HITECH Act in addition to complying with HIPAA. The solution is particularly useful for independent physician practices with less than 10 physicians.

9.2.2 Subject of the case-study

This case study involves 45 independent physician practices in Newport Beach California, many of them with 1–2 physicians. There is a total of 145 users (physicians, nurse practitioners and office staff). Users come from multiple specialties including— pulmonary, neurosurgery, internal medicine, nephrology, vascular surgery, thoracic surgery, and cardiology.

9.2.3 *Selection*

Mitochon Systems was chosen by these physicians primarily because of the low cost, comprehensive HIE functionality, and ease of use. Single physician and small office practices often cited the lack of in-house IT personnel or expertise to manage an in-house infrastructure as an impediment to adopting an EMR solution. Mitochon's Cloud solution therefore made sense to them. With this web-based solution, physicians were able to access all the functionality they needed, but did not have to worry about the underlying technology issues. In the Mitochon Cloud-based system, all information is stored in a HIPAA compliant manner with Amazon EC2 cloud. This is a highly secure environment and all data is encrypted. The security of the Cloud-based solution was underlined when two physician offices reported instances of theft—leading to Laptops and computers being stolen. However, because patient information was stored in the cloud and not in-house, there was no breach of security and no patient information was lost.

9.2.4 Getting started

Obtaining an account with Mitochon is similar to obtaining an account with any online web-portal. Subscribers can go the company website and apply for an account. The registration process can be accomplished in minutes. Within 24 hours, Mitochon verifies the information, calls the subscriber in order to validate the information and activates the account.

9.2.5 Training

The training on the system is mainly via webinars and runs into several hours for a typical practice. Follow-up training is occasionally required. On-site training has been requested in remarkably few cases and web-based training normally suffices.

9.2.6 Paper to digital conversion

This is the most labor intensive and onerous step, as viewed by new users of EMR systems. Digital conversion of earlier paper-based records is however essential. The degree of effort required to digitize legacy data is directly proportional to how long the physician has been practicing. This puts younger doctors at a distinct advantage when it comes to digitization of earlier records. The recommended strategy is for the office staff to only scan and digitally convert the charts of patients who are scheduled for appointments in the next 1–2 weeks. Over approximately a 12 month period, all the charts are typically converted. This process results in minimal disruption. The physicians noted that in the 1–2 week period immediately following the adoption of the system, a typical patient visit often took about twice the time as it did earlier because the physicians had to validate and add additional information such as allergy information, past medications, etc. This problem does not arise on subsequent visits due to the system's ability to efficiently retrieve this information.

The physicians can directly dictate into the application using Dragon Medical speech recognition software. They can also build their own personal library of templates personalized for easy capture of information which improves documentation compliance.

9.2.7 Workflow changes

The changes noted by the physicians who transition from a paper-based system mainly relate to the fact that the computer is now in the physician's room. As noted by users of other EMR systems, physicians end up dividing their time between the patient and the EMR system. Mitochon's solution allows the physician to use hand writing recognition technology and voice recognition technology in addition to simply typing information. In addition the solution allows for template customization and creation by the user. The physical exam template allows the creation of customized specialty-specific findings. The templates for the "assessment section" allow for the creation of customized, disease/illness specific treatment plans. Majority of physicians either dictate the entire encounter, or use a "cloning" function to copy forward the data from prior visits and then augment the document to reflect the new findings and plans.

9.2.8 Cloud Specific Benefits

Integrated HIE

The HIE integration was noted to be of most value to small practices. Most small practices spend an inordinate amount of time gathering information from other physicians. This Cloud solution allows any network member of the virtual medical community to access and share problems list, medication list, progress notes etc with other members in a HIPAA compliant manner. What would have earlier taken up to an hour is now done in minutes. Also once the information is in the system, there is no need to repeat scanning, because the information is automatically indexed and presented to the physicians for orderly viewing. The system has been used to exchange tens of thousands of files to-date.

Propagation of updates/enhancements

Because of the inevitable enhancements and upgrades that will be needed to meet "meaningful use" and changing healthcare guidelines, ease of system upgrades will be key feature for all EMR systems. Because the Mitochon system is Cloud-based, users do not have to worry about these upgrades at all. On average, Mitochon adds between 50–80 enhancements every 3 months.

Integration

Integration is made easier because Mitochon has published its web services. e-prescribing functionality is integrated with H2H ePrescription. "Clinical Groupware", is a concept pioneered by David Kibbe, MD in which many Cloud-based applications can be quickly integrated to create a portfolio of functionality desired by the user. Mitochon supports such a concept because it can quickly and easily integrate with offerings from other HIT vendors.

Electronic Prescription

Mitochon's Cloud solution with integrated HIE architecture allows all network users to have separate but identical medication lists. In this network, after the initial medication list is confirmed as active by the first physician on a particular patient chart, subsequent additional electronic prescription changes made by any other physician automatically update the medication list of all physician users on the network who are providing care to the particular patient.

9.2.8 Summary

The Mitochon Virtual Medical Community of 45 physicians, which is the subject of this case study has been in successful operation since February 2009. Mitochon continually upgrades its web-based offering to comply with Meaningful Use criteria as they are released.

APPENDICES

HIPAA Security Checklist

HIPAA Security Rule Reference	Safeguard	(R) = Required, (A) = Addressable
Administrative Safeguards		
164.308(a)(1)(i)	Security management process: Implement policies and procedures to prevent, detect, contain, and correct security violations.	
164.308(a)(1)(ii)(A)	Has a risk analysis been completed IAW NIST using Guidelines?	(R)
164.308(a)(1)(ii)(B)	Has the risk management process been completed using IAW NIST Guidelines?	(R)
164.308(a)(1)(ii)(C)	Do you have formal sanctions against employees who fail to comply with security policies and procedures?	(R)
164.308(a)(1)(ii)(D)	Have you implemented procedures to regularly review records of IS activity such as audit logs, access reports, and security incident tracking?	(R)
164.308(a)(2)	Assigned security responsibility: Identify the security official who is responsible for the development and implementation of the policies and procedures required by this subpart for the entity.	
164.308(a)(3)(i)	Workforce security: Implement policies and procedures to ensure that all members of workforce have appropriate access to EPHI, as provided under paragraph (a)(4) of this section, and to prevent those workforce members who do not have access under paragraph (a)	

Appendix A contd...

Appendix A contd...

HIPAA Security Rule Reference	Safeguard	(R) = Required, (A) = Addressable
Administrative Safeguards		
	(4) of this section from obtaining access to electronic protected health information (EPHI).	
164.308(a)(3)(ii)(A)	Have you implemented procedures for the authorization and/or supervision of employees who work with EPHI or in locations where it might be accessed?	(A)
164.308(a)(3)(ii)(B)	Have you implemented procedures to determine the access of an employee to EPHI is appropriate?	(A)
164.308(a)(3)(ii)(C)	Have you implemented procedures for terminating access to EPHI when an employee leaves your organization or as required by paragraph (a)(3)(ii)(B) of this section?	(A)
164.308(a)(4)(i)	Information access management: Implement policies and procedures for authorizing access to EPHI that are consistent with the applicable requirements of subpart E of this part.	
164.308(a)(4)(ii)(A)	If you are a clearinghouse that is part of a larger organization, have you implemented policies and procedures to protect EPHI from the larger organization?	(A)
164.308(a)(4)(ii)(B)	Have you implemented policies and procedures for granting access to EPHI, for example, through access to a workstation, transaction, program, or process?	(A)
164.308(a)(4)(ii)(C)	Have you implemented policies and procedures that are based upon your access authorization policies, established, document, review, and modify a user's right of access to a workstation, transaction, program, or process?	(A)

HIPAA Security Rule Reference	Safeguard	(R) = Required, (A) = Addressable
Administrative Safeguards		
164.308(a)(5)(i)	Security awareness and training: Implement a security awareness and training program for all members of the workforce (including management).	
164.308(a)(5)(ii)(A)	Do you provide periodic information security reminders?	(A)
164.308(a)(5)(ii)(B)	Do you have policies and procedures for guarding against, detecting, and reporting malicious software?	(A)
164.308(a)(5)(ii)(C)	Do you have procedures for monitoring log-in attempts and reporting discrepancies?	(A)
164.308(a)(5)(ii)(D)	Do you have procedures for creating, changing, and safeguarding passwords?	(A)
164.308(a)(6)(i)	Security incident procedures: Implement policies and procedures to address security incidents.	
164.308(a)(6)(ii)	Do you have procedures to identify and respond to suspected or known security incidents; to mitigate them to the extent practicable, measure harmful effects of known security incidents; and document incidents and their outcomes?	(R)
164.308(a)(7)(i)	Contingency plan: Establish (and implement as needed) policies and procedures for responding to an emergency or other occurrence (for example, fire, vandalism, system failure, or natural disaster) that damages systems that contain EPHI. 164.308(a)(7)(ii)(A) Have you established and implemented procedures to create and maintain retrievable exact copies of EPHI?	(R)

Appendix A contd...

Appendix A contd...

HIPAA Security Rule Reference	Safeguard	(R) = Required, (A) = Addressable
Administrative Safeguards		
164.308(a)(7)(ii)(B)	Have you established (and implemented as needed) procedures to restore any loss of EPHI data stored electronically?	(R)
164.308(a)(7)(ii)(C)	Have you established (and implemented as needed) procedures to enable continuation of critical business processes and for protection of EPHI while operating in the emergency mode?	(R)
164.308(a)(7)(ii)(D)	Have you implemented procedures for periodic testing and revision of contingency plans?	(A)
164.308(a)(7)(ii)(E)	Have you assessed the relative criticality of specific applications and data in support of other contingency plan components?	(A)
164.308(a)(8)	Have you established a plan for periodic technical and nontechnical evaluation, based initially upon the standards implemented under this rule and subsequently, in response to environmental or operational changes affecting the security of EPHI, that establishes the extent to which an entity's security policies and procedures meet the requirements of this subpart?	(R)
164.308(b)(1)	Business associate contracts and other arrangements: A covered entity, in accordance with Sec. 164.306, may permit a business associate to create, receive, maintain, or transmit EPHI on the covered entity's behalf only if the covered entity obtains satisfactory assurances in accordance with Sec. 164.314(a) that the business associate appropriately safeguards the information.	

HIPAA Security Rule Reference	Safeguard	(R) = Required, (A) = Addressable
Administrative Safeguards		
164.308(b)(4)	Have you established written contracts or other arrangements with your trading partners that document satisfactory assurances required by paragraph (b)(1) of this section that meets the applicable requirements of Sec. 164.314(a)?	(R)
Physical Safeguards		
164.310(a)(1)	Facility access controls: Implement policies and procedures to limit physical access to electronic information systems and the facility or facilities in which they are housed, while ensuring properly authorized access is allowed.	
164.310(a)(2)(i)	Have you established (and implemented as needed) procedures that allow facility access in support of restoration of lost data under the disaster recovery plan and emergency mode operations plan?	(A)
164.310(a)(2)(ii)	Have you implemented policies and procedures to safeguard the facility and the equipment therein from unauthorized physical access, tampering, and theft?	(A)
164.310(a)(2)(iii)	Have you implemented procedures to control and validate a person's access to facilities based on his/her role or function, including visitor control, and control of access to software programs for testing and revision?	(A)
164.310(a)(2)(iv)	Have you implemented policies and procedures to document repairs and modifications to the physical components of a facility that are related to security (for example, hardware, walls, doors, and locks)?	(A)

Appendix A contd...

Appendix A contd...

HIPAA Security Rule Reference	Safeguard	(R) = Required, (A) = Addressable
Physical Safeguards		
164.310(b)	Have you implemented policies and procedures that specify the proper functions to be performed, the manner in which those functions are to be performed, and the physical attributes of the surroundings of a specific workstation or class of workstation that can access EPHI?	(R)
164.310(c)	Have you implemented physical safeguards for all workstations that access EPHI to restrict access to authorized users?	(R)
164.310(d)(1)	Device and media controls: Implement policies and procedures that govern the receipt and removal of hardware and electronic media that contain EPHI into and out of a facility, and the movement of these items within the facility.	
164.310(d)(2)(i)	Have you implemented policies and procedures to address final disposition of EPHI, and/or hardware or electronic media on which it is stored?	(R)
164.310(d)(2)(ii)	Have you implemented procedures for removal of EPHI from electronic media before the media are available for reuse?	(R)
164.310(d)(2)(iii)	Do you maintain a record of the movements of hardware and electronic media and the person responsible for its movement?	(A)
164.310(d)(2)(iv)	Do you create a retrievable, exact copy of EPHI, when needed, before moving equipment?	(A)
164.312(a)(1)	Access controls: Implement technical policies and procedures for electronic information systems that maintain EPHI to allow access only to those	

HIPAA Security Rule Reference	Safeguard	(R) = Required, (A) = Addressable
Technical Safeguards		
	persons or software programs that have been granted access rights as specified in Sec. 164.308(a)(4).	
164.312(a)(2)(i)	Have you assigned a unique name and/or number for identifying and tracking user identity?	(R)
164.312(a)(2)(ii)	Have you established (and implemented as needed) procedures for obtaining necessary EPHI during an emergency?	(R)
164.312(a)(2)(iii)	Have you implemented procedures that terminate an electronic session after a predetermined time of inactivity?	(A)
164.312(a)(2)(iv)	Have you implemented a mechanism to encrypt and decrypt EPHI?	(A)
164.312(b)	Have you implemented audit controls, hardware, software, and/or procedural mechanisms that record and examine activity in information systems that contain or use EPHI?	(R)
164.312(c)(1)	Integrity: Implement policies and procedures to protect EPHI from improper alteration or destruction.	
164.312(c)(2)	Have you implemented electronic mechanisms to corroborate that EPHI has not been altered or destroyed in an unauthorized manner?	(A)
164.312(d)	Have you implemented person or entity authentication procedures to verify a person or entity seeking access EPHI is the one claimed?	(R)
164.312(e)(1)	Transmission security: Implement technical security measures to guard against unauthorized access to EPHI being transmitted over an electronic communications network.	

Appendix A contd...

Appendix A contd...

HIPAA Security Rule Reference	Safeguard	(R) = Required, (A) = Addressable
Technical Safeguards		
164.312(e)(2)(i)	Have you implemented security measures to ensure electronically transmitted EPHI is not improperly modified without detection until disposed of?	(A)
164.312(e)(2)(ii)	Have you implemented a mechanism to encrypt EPHI whenever deemed appropriate?	(A)

Sample Business Associate Contract

This contract is provided by HHS on its website at the following location: [http://www.hhs.gov/ocr/privacy/hipaa/understanding/coveredentities/contractprov.html]

BUSINESS ASSOCIATE CONTRACT SAMPLE

Definitions (alternative approaches)

Catch-all definition:

Terms used, but not otherwise defined, in this Agreement shall have the same meaning as those terms in the Privacy Rule.

Examples of specific definitions:

   a. Business Associate. "Business Associate" shall mean [Insert Name of Business Associate].
   b. Covered Entity. "Covered Entity" shall mean [Insert Name of Covered Entity].
   c. Individual. "Individual" shall have the same meaning as the term "individual" in 45 CFR 160.103 and shall include a person who qualifies as a personal representative in accordance with 45 CFR 164.502(g).
   d. Privacy Rule. "Privacy Rule" shall mean the Standards for Privacy of Individually Identifiable Health Information at 45 CFR Part 160 and Part 164, Subparts A and E.
   e. Protected Health Information. "Protected Health Information" shall have the same meaning as the term "protected health information" in 45 CFR 160.103, limited to the information created or received by Business Associate from or on behalf of Covered Entity.

f. Required By Law. "Required By Law" shall have the same meaning as the term "required by law" in 45 CFR 164.103.

g. Secretary. "Secretary" shall mean the Secretary of the Department of Health and Human Services or his designee.

Obligations and Activities of Business Associate

a. Business Associate agrees to not use or disclose Protected Health Information other than as permitted or required by the Agreement or as Required By Law.

b. Business Associate agrees to use appropriate safeguards to prevent use or disclosure of the Protected Health Information other than as provided for by this Agreement.

c. Business Associate agrees to mitigate, to the extent practicable, any harmful effect that is known to Business Associate of a use or disclosure of Protected Health Information by Business Associate in violation of the requirements of this Agreement. [This provision may be included if it is appropriate for the Covered Entity to pass on its duty to mitigate damages to a Business Associate].

d. Business Associate agrees to report to Covered Entity any use or disclosure of the Protected Health Information not provided for by this Agreement of which it becomes aware.

e. Business Associate agrees to ensure that any agent, including a subcontractor, to whom it provides Protected Health Information received from, or created or received by Business Associate on behalf of Covered Entity agrees to the same restrictions and conditions that apply through this Agreement to Business Associate with respect to such information.

f. Business Associate agrees to provide access, at the request of Covered Entity, and in the time and manner [Insert negotiated terms], to Protected Health Information in a Designated Record Set, to Covered Entity or, as directed by Covered Entity, to an Individual in order to meet the requirements under 45 CFR 164.524. [Not necessary if business associate does not have protected health information in a designated record set].

g. Business Associate agrees to make any amendment(s) to Protected Health Information in a Designated Record Set that the Covered Entity directs or agrees to pursuant to 45

CFR 164.526 at the request of Covered Entity or an Individual, and in the time and manner [Insert negotiated terms]. [Not necessary if business associate does not have protected health information in a designated record set].

h. Business Associate agrees to make internal practices, books, and records, including policies and procedures and Protected Health Information, relating to the use and disclosure of Protected Health Information received from, or created or received by Business Associate on behalf of, Covered Entity available [to the Covered Entity, or] to the Secretary, in a time and manner [Insert negotiated terms] or designated by the Secretary, for purposes of the Secretary determining Covered Entity's compliance with the Privacy Rule.

i. Business Associate agrees to document such disclosures of Protected Health Information and information related to such disclosures as would be required for Covered Entity to respond to a request by an Individual for an accounting of disclosures of Protected Health Information in accordance with 45 CFR 164.528.

j. Business Associate agrees to provide to Covered Entity or an Individual, in time and manner [Insert negotiated terms], information collected in accordance with Section [Insert Section Number in Contract Where Provision (i) Appears] of this Agreement, to permit Covered Entity to respond to a request by an Individual for an accounting of disclosures of Protected Health Information in accordance with 45 CFR 164.528.

Permitted Uses and Disclosures by Business Associate

General Use and Disclosure Provisions [(a) and (b) are alternative approaches]

a. *Specify purposes:*
   Except as otherwise limited in this Agreement, Business Associate may use or disclose Protected Health Information on behalf of, or to provide services to, Covered Entity for the following purposes, if such use or disclosure of Protected Health Information would not violate the Privacy Rule if done by Covered Entity or the minimum necessary policies and procedures of the Covered Entity: [List Purposes].

b. *Refer to underlying services agreement:*

Except as otherwise limited in this Agreement, Business Associate may use or disclose Protected Health Information to perform functions, activities, or services for, or on behalf of, Covered Entity as specified in [Insert Name of Services Agreement], provided that such use or disclosure would not violate the Privacy Rule if done by Covered Entity or the minimum necessary policies and procedures of the Covered Entity.

Specific Use and Disclosure Provisions [only necessary if parties wish to allow Business Associate to engage in such activities]

a. Except as otherwise limited in this Agreement, Business Associate may use Protected Health Information for the proper management and administration of the Business Associate or to carry out the legal responsibilities of the Business Associate.

b. Except as otherwise limited in this Agreement, Business Associate may disclose Protected Health Information for the proper management and administration of the Business Associate, provided that disclosures are Required By Law, or Business Associate obtains reasonable assurances from the person to whom the information is disclosed that it will remain confidential and used or further disclosed only as Required By Law or for the purpose for which it was disclosed to the person, and the person notifies the Business Associate of any instances of which it is aware in which the confidentiality of the information has been breached.

c. Except as otherwise limited in this Agreement, Business Associate may use Protected Health Information to provide Data Aggregation services to Covered Entity as permitted by 45 CFR 164.504(e)(2)(i)(B).

d. Business Associate may use Protected Health Information to report violations of law to appropriate Federal and State authorities, consistent with 164.502(j)(1).

Obligations of Covered Entity

Provisions for Covered Entity to Inform Business Associate of Privacy Practices and Restrictions [provisions dependent on business arrangement]

a. Covered Entity shall notify Business Associate of any limitation(s) in its notice of privacy practices of Covered Entity in accordance with 45 CFR 164.520, to the extent that such limitation may affect Business Associate's use or disclosure of Protected Health Information.

b. Covered Entity shall notify Business Associate of any changes in, or revocation of, permission by Individual to use or disclose Protected Health Information, to the extent that such changes may affect Business Associate's use or disclosure of Protected Health Information.

c. Covered Entity shall notify Business Associate of any restriction to the use or disclosure of Protected Health Information that Covered Entity has agreed to in accordance with 45 CFR 164.522, to the extent that such restriction may affect Business Associate's use or disclosure of Protected Health Information.

Permissible Requests by Covered Entity

Covered Entity shall not request Business Associate to use or disclose Protected Health Information in any manner that would not be permissible under the Privacy Rule if done by Covered Entity. [Include an exception if the Business Associate will use or disclose protected health information for, and the contract includes provisions for, data aggregation or management and administrative activities of Business Associate].

Term and Termination

a. Term. The Term of this Agreement shall be effective as of [Insert Effective Date], and shall terminate when all of the Protected Health Information provided by Covered Entity to Business Associate, or created or received by Business Associate on behalf of Covered Entity, is destroyed or returned to Covered Entity, or, if it is infeasible to return or destroy Protected Health Information, protections are extended to such information, in accordance with the termination provisions in this Section. [Term may differ.]

b. Termination for Cause. Upon Covered Entity's knowledge of a material breach by Business Associate, Covered Entity shall either:

1. Provide an opportunity for Business Associate to cure the breach or end the violation and terminate this Agreement [and the _____ Agreement/sections ____ of the _____ Agreement] if Business Associate does not cure the breach or end the violation within the time specified by Covered Entity;

2. Immediately terminate this Agreement [and the _____ Agreement/sections ____ of the _____ Agreement] if Business Associate has breached a material term of this Agreement and cure is not possible; or

3. If neither termination nor cure are feasible, Covered Entity shall report the violation to the Secretary.

   [Bracketed language in this provision may be necessary if there is an underlying services agreement. Also, opportunity to cure is permitted, but not required by the Privacy Rule].

C. *Effect of Termination.*

1. Except as provided in paragraph (2) of this section, upon termination of this Agreement, for any reason, Business Associate shall return or destroy all Protected Health Information received from Covered Entity, or created or received by Business Associate on behalf of Covered Entity. This provision shall apply to Protected Health Information that is in the possession of subcontractors or agents of Business Associate. Business Associate shall retain no copies of the Protected Health Information.

2. In the event that Business Associate determines that returning or destroying the Protected Health Information is infeasible, Business Associate shall provide to Covered Entity notification of the conditions that make return or destruction infeasible. Upon [Insert negotiated terms] that return or destruction of Protected Health Information is infeasible, Business Associate shall extend the protections of this Agreement to such Protected Health Information and limit further uses and disclosures of such Protected Health Information to those purposes that make the return or destruction infeasible, for so long as Business Associate maintains such Protected Health Information.

Miscellaneous

a. Regulatory References. A reference in this Agreement to a section in the Privacy Rule means the section as in effect or as amended.

b. Amendment. The Parties agree to take such action as is necessary to amend this Agreement from time to time as is necessary for Covered Entity to comply with the requirements of the Privacy Rule and the Health Insurance Portability and Accountability Act of 1996, Pub. L. No. 104–191.

c. Survival. The respective rights and obligations of Business Associate under Section [Insert Section Number Related to "Effect of Termination"] of this Agreement shall survive the termination of this Agreement.

d. Interpretation. Any ambiguity in this Agreement shall be resolved to permit Covered Entity to comply with the Privacy Rule.

Meaningful Use Guidelines and Certification Criteria

The following table summarizes the Objectives for "meaningful use" for Stage I, and the measure used to verify compliance in each case. The third column shows the relevant certification criteria for the EHR system. This information is extracted from the DHHS document at [http://www.ofr.gov/OFRUpload/OFRData/2010-17210_PI.pdf].

CORE OBJECTIVES		
Objective	Measure	Certification Criteria
Use CPOE for medication orders directly entered by any licensed healthcare professional who can enter orders into the medical record per state, local and professional guidelines.	More than 30% of unique patients with at least one medication in their medication list seen by the EP or admitted to the eligible hospital's or CAH's inpatient or emergency department have at least one medication order entered using CPOE.	Enable a user to electronically record, store, retrieve, and modify, at a minimum, the following order types: (1) Medications; (2) Laboratory; and (3) Radiology/imaging.
Implement drug-drug and drug-allergy interaction checks.	Functionality is enabled for the entire reporting period for these checks.	(1) Notifications. Automatically and electronically generate and indicate in real-time, notifications at the point of care for drug-drug and drug-allergy contraindications based on medication list, medication allergy list, and computerized provider order entry (CPOE).

Appendix C contd...

Appendix C contd...

CORE OBJECTIVES

Objective	Measure	Certification Criteria
		(2) <u>Adjustments</u>. Provide certain users with the ability to adjust notifications provided for drug-drug and drug-allergy interaction checks.
Generate and transmit permissible prescriptions electronically.	More than 40% of all permissible prescriptions written by the EP are transmitted electronically using certified EHR technology.	Electronic prescribing. Enable a user to electronically generate and transmit prescriptions and prescription-related information in accordance with relevant standards.
Record patient demographics (sex, race, ethnicity, date of birth, preferred language, and in the case of hospitals, date and preliminary cause of death in the event of mortality).	More than 50 percent of patients' demographic data to be recorded as structured data.	Enable a user to electronically record, modify, and retrieve patient demographic data including preferred language, gender, race, ethnicity, and date of birth. Enable race and ethnicity to be recorded in accordance with the standard specified at 170.207(f).
Maintain up-to-date problem list of current and active diagnoses.	More than 80% of all unique patients seen by the EP or admitted to the eligible hospital's or CAH's inpatient or emergency department have at least one entry or an indication that no problems are known for the patient recorded as structured data.	Maintain up-to-date problem list. Enable a user to electronically record, modify, and retrieve a patient's problem list for longitudinal care.

Appendix C contd...

CORE OBJECTIVES		
Objective	**Measure**	**Certification Criteria**
Maintain active medication list	More than 80% of all unique patients seen by the EP or admitted to the eligible hospital's or CAH's inpatient or emergency department have at least one entry (or an indication that the patient is not currently prescribed any medication) recorded as structured data.	Maintain active medication list. Enable a user to electronically record, modify, and retrieve a patient's active medication list as well as medication history for longitudinal care.
Maintain active medication allergy list	More than 80% of all unique patients seen by the EP or admitted to the eligible hospital's or CAH's inpatient or emergency department have at least one entry (or an indication that the patient has no known medication allergies) recorded as structured data.	Enable a user to electronically record, modify, and retrieve a patient's active medication allergy list as well as medication allergy history for longitudinal care.
Record and chart changes in vital signs: • Height • Weight • Blood pressure • Calculate and display BMI • Plot and display growth charts for children 2–20 years, including BMI.	For more than 50% of all unique patients age 2 and over seen by the EP or admitted to eligible hospital's or CAH's inpatient or emergency department, height, weight and blood pressure are recorded as structured data.	(1)Vital signs. Enable a user to electronically record, modify, and retrieve a patient's vital signs including, at a minimum, height, weight, and blood pressure. (2)Calculate body mass index. Automatically calculate and display body mass index (BMI) based on a patient's height and weight. (3) Plot and display growth charts. Plot and electronically display, upon request, growth charts for patients 2–20 years old.

CORE OBJECTIVES		
Objective	**Measure**	**Certification Criteria**
Record smoking status for patients 13 years of age of older.	More than 50% of all unique patients 13 years old or older seen by the EP or admitted to the eligible hospital's or CAH's inpatient or emergency department have smoking status recorded as structured data.	Enable a user to electronically record, modify, and retrieve the smoking status of a patient. Smoking status types must include: current every day smoker; current some day smoker; former smoker; never smoker; smoker, current status unknown; and unknown if ever smoked.
Implement one clinical decision support rule and ability to track compliance with the rule.	One clinical decision support rule implemented.	Implement automated, electronic clinical decision support rules (in addition to drug-drug and drug allergy contraindication checking) based on the data elements included in: problem list; medication list; demographics; and laboratory test results. Automatically and electronically generate and indicate in real-time, notifications and care suggestions based upon clinical decision support rules.

Appendix C contd...

Appendix C contd...

CORE OBJECTIVES		
Objective	**Measure**	**Certification Criteria**
Eligible Professionals: Report ambulatory clinical quality measures to CMS or the States Eligible Hospitals and CAHs: Report hospital clinical quality measures to CMS or the States.	For 2011, provide aggregate numerator, denominator, and exclusions through attestation. For 2012, electronically submit the clinical quality measures.	(1) Calculate. (i) Electronically calculate all of the core clinical measures specified by CMS for eligible professionals. (ii) Electronically calculate, at a minimum, three clinical quality measures specified by CMS for eligible professionals, in addition to those clinical quality measures specified. (2) Submission. Enable a user to electronically submit calculated clinical quality measures in accordance with the standard and implementation specifications Electronically calculate all of the clinical quality measures specified by CMS for eligible hospitals and critical access hospitals. Enable a user to electronically submit calculated clinical quality measures in accordance with the standard and implementation specifications specified.

CORE OBJECTIVES		
Objective	**Measure**	**Certification Criteria**
On request, provide patients with an electronic copy of their health information (including diagnostic test results, problem list, medication list, medication allergies, and for hospitals, discharge summary and procedures).	More than 50% of all patients of the EP or the inpatient or emergency departments of the eligible hospital or CAH who request an electronic copy of their health information are provided it within 3 business days.	Enable a user to create an electronic copy of a patient's clinical information, including, at a minimum, diagnostic test results, problem list, medication list, and medication allergy list in: (1) Human readable format; and (2) On electronic media or through some other electronic means in accordance in accordance with relevant standards and applicable implementations for Problems, Laboratory Test Results and Medications.
Provide clinical summaries for patients for each office visit.	Clinical summaries provided to patients for more than 50% of all office visits within 3 business days.	Enable a user to provide clinical summaries to patients for each office visit that include, at a minimum, diagnostic test results, problem list, medication list, and medication allergy list. If the clinical summary is provided electronically it must be: (1) Provided in human readable format; and (2) Provided on electronic media or through some other electronic means.

Appendix C contd...

Appendix C contd...

CORE OBJECTIVES		
Objective	**Measure**	**Certification Criteria**
		in accordance with relevant standards and applicable implementations for Problems, Laboratory Test Results and Medications.
Capability to exchange key clinical information (for example, problem list, medication list, medication allergies, diagnostic test results), among providers of care and patient authorized entities electronically The EP, eligible hospital or CAH who transitions their patient to another setting of care or provider of care or refers their patient to another provider of care should provide summary of care record for each transition of care or referral.	Performed at least one test of certified EHR technology's capacity to electronically exchange key clinical information ---------------------- The EP, eligible hospital or CAH who transitions or refers their patient to another setting of care or provider of care provides a summary of care record for more than 50% of transitions of care and referrals.	Electronically receive and display a patient's summary record, from other providers and organizations including, at a minimum, diagnostic tests results, problem list, medication list, and medication allergy list in accordance with the standard and applicable implementation specifications. Upon receipt of a patient summary record formatted according to the alternative standard, display it in human readable format. Enable a user to electronically transmit a patient summary record to other providers and organizations including, at a minimum, diagnostic test results, problem list, medication list, and medication allergy list in accordance with relevant standards and implementation specifications.

CORE OBJECTIVES		
Objective	**Measure**	**Certification Criteria**
Protect electronic health information created or maintained by the certified EHR technology through the implementation of appropriate technical capabilities.	Conduct or review a security risk analysis and implement security updates as necessary and correct identified security deficiencies as part of its risk management process.	Access control. Assign a unique name and/or number for identifying and tracking user identity and establish controls that permit only authorized users to access electronic health information. Emergency access. Permit authorized users (who are authorized for emergency situations) to access electronic health information during an emergency. Automatic log-off. Terminate an electronic session after a predetermined time of inactivity. Record actions. Record actions related to electronic health information in accordance with the standard specified. Generate audit log. Enable a user to generate an audit log for a specific time period and to sort entries in the audit log according to any of the elements specified in the standard. (1) Create a message digest in accordance with the standard specified.

Appendix C contd...

Appendix C contd...

CORE OBJECTIVES		
Objective	**Measure**	**Certification Criteria**
		(2) Verify in accordance with the standard specified upon receipt of electronically exchanged health information that such information has not been altered. (3) Detection. Detect the alteration of audit logs. Verify that a person or entity seeking access to electronic health information is the one claimed and is authorized to access such information. Encrypt and decrypt electronic health information in accordance with the standard specified, unless the Secretary determines that the use of such algorithm would pose a significant security risk for Certified EHR Technology. Encrypt and decrypt electronic health information when exchanged in accordance with the standard specified. Record disclosures made for treatment, payment, and health care operations in accordance with the standard specified.

CORE OBJECTIVES		
MENU		
Implement drug formulary checks.	Drug formulary check system is enabled and provider has access to at least one internal or external drug formulary for the entire reporting period.	Enable a user to electronically check if drugs are in a formulary or preferred drug list.
Record advance directives for patients 65 years of age or older. (Applies to hospitals only).	More than 50% of all unique patients 65 years old or older admitted to the eligible hospital's or CAH's inpatient department have an indication of an advance directive status recorded.	Enable a user to electronically record whether a patient has an advance directive.
Incorporate clinical laboratory test results into EHRs as structured data.	More than 40% of all clinical lab tests results ordered by the EP or by an authorized provider of the eligible hospital or CAH for patients admitted to its inpatient or emergency department during the HER reporting period whose results are either in a positive/negative or numerical format are incorporated in certified HER technology as structured data.	(1) Electronically receive clinical laboratory test results in a structured format and display such results in human readable format. (2) Display test report information. (3) Incorporate results. Electronically attribute, associate, or link a laboratory test result to a laboratory order or patient record.
Generate lists of patients by specific conditions to use for quality improvement, reduction of disparities, research or outreach	Generate at least one listing of patients with specific condition	Generate patient lists. Enable a user to electronically select, sort, retrieve, and generate lists of patients according to, at a minimum, the data elements included in:

Appendix C contd...

Appendix C contd...

CORE OBJECTIVES		
Objective	**Measure**	**Certification Criteria**
MENU		
		(1) Problem list; (2) Medication list; (3) Demographics; and (4) Laboratory test results.
Send reminders to patients per patient preference for preventive/follow up care. (For Eligible Providers only)	More than 20% of all unique patients 65 years or older or 5 years old or younger were sent an appropriate reminder during the EHR reporting period	Enable a user to electronically generate a patient reminder list for preventive or follow-up care according to patient preferences based on, at a minimum, the data elements included in: (1) Problem list; (2) Medication list; (3) Medication allergy list; (4) Demographics; and (5) Laboratory test results.
Provide patients with timely electronic access to their health information (including laboratory results, problem list, medication lists, medication allergies) —Applies to Eligible Professionals only.	More than 10 percent of patients are provided electronic access to information within four days of it being updated in the EHR.	Enable a user to provide patients with online access to their clinical information, including, at a minimum, lab test results, problem list, medication list, and medication allergy list.
Use certified EHR technology to identify patient-specific education resources and provide those resources to the patient if appropriate.	More than 10% of all unique patients seen by the EP or admitted to the eligible hospital's or CAH's inpatient or emergency department are provided patient-specific education resources	Patient-specific education resources. Enable a user to electronically identify and provide patient-specific education resources according to, at a minimum, the data elements included in

CORE OBJECTIVES		
Objective	**Measure**	**Certification Criteria**
MENU		
		the patient's: problem list; medication list; and laboratory test results; as well as provide such resources to the patient.
The EP, eligible hospital or CAH who receives a patient from another setting of care or provider of care or believes an encounter is relevant should perform medication reconciliation.	The EP, eligible hospital or CAH performs medication reconciliation for more than 50% of transitions of care in which the patient is transitioned into the care of the EP or admitted to the eligible hospital's or CAH's inpatient or emergency department.	Medication reconciliation. Enable a user to electronically compare two or more medication lists.
The EP, eligible hospital or CAH who transitions their patient to another setting of care or provider of care or refers their patient to another provider of care should provide summary of care record for each transition of care or referral.	Summary of care record is provided for more than 50 percent of patient transitions or referrals.	
Capability to submit electronic data to immunization registries or Immunization Information Systems and actual submission in accordance with applicable law and practice.	Performed at least one test of certified EHR technology's capacity to submit electronic data to immunization registries and follow up submission if the test is successful (unless none of the immunization registries to which the EP, eligible hospital	Electronically record, modify, retrieve, and submit immunization information in accordance with appropriate standards and specifications.

Appendix C contd...

Appendix C contd...

CORE OBJECTIVES		
Objective	**Measure**	**Certification Criteria**
MENU		
	or CAH submits such information have the capacity to receive the information electronically).	
Capability to submit electronic data on reportable (as required by state or local law) lab results to public health agencies and actual submission in accordance with applicable law and practice. (Applicable for hospitals & CAH only).	Performed at least one test of certified EHR technology's capacity to provide electronic submission of reportable lab results to public health agencies and follow-up submission if the test is successful (unless none of the public health agencies to which eligible hospital or CAH submits such information have the capacity to receive the information electronically).	Electronically record, modify, retrieve, and submit reportable clinical lab results in accordance with the standard (and applicable implementation specifications).
Capability to submit electronic syndromic surveillance data to public health agencies and actual submission in accordance with applicable law and practice.	Performed at least one test of certified EHR technology's capacity to provide electronic syndromic surveillance data to public health agencies and follow-up submission if the test is successful (unless none of the public health agencies to which an EP, eligible hospital or CAH submits such information have the capacity to receive the information electronically).	Electronically record, modify, retrieve, and submit syndrome-based public health surveillance information in accordance with the standard and applicable implementation specifications.

Sample — Interview and Document Request for HIPAA Security Onsite Investigations and Compliance Reviews

This is a DHHS/CMS Document released by the Office of E-Health Standards and Services

1. Personnel that may be interviewed
   - President, CEO or Director
   - HIPAA Compliance Officer
   - Lead Systems Manager or Director
   - Systems Security Officer
   - Lead Network Engineer and/or individuals responsible for:
     o administration of systems which store, transmit, or access Electronic Protected Health Information (EPHI)
     o administration systems networks (wired and wireless)
     o monitoring of systems which store, transmit, or access EPHI
     o monitoring systems networks (if different from above)
   - Computer Hardware Specialist
   - Disaster Recovery Specialist or person in charge of data backup
   - Facility Access Control Coordinator (physical security)
   - Human Resources Representative
   - Director of Training
   - Incident Response Team Leader
   - Others as identified….

2. Documents and other information that may be requested for investigations/reviews

   a. Policies and Procedures and other Evidence that Address the Following:

   - Prevention, detection, containment, and correction of security violations
   - Employee background checks and confidentiality agreements
   - Establishing user access for new and existing employees
   - List of authentication methods used to identify users authorized to access EPHI
   - List of individuals and contractors with access to EPHI to include copies pertinent business associate agreements
   - List of software used to manage and control access to the Internet
   - Detecting, reporting, and responding to security incidents (if not in the security plan)
   - Physical security
   - Encryption and decryption of EPHI
   - Mechanisms to ensure integrity of data during transmission —including portable media transmission (i.e., laptops, cell phones, blackberries, thumb drives)
   - Monitoring systems use—authorized and unauthorized
   - Use of wireless networks
   - Granting, approving, and monitoring systems access (for example, by level, role, and job function)
   - Sanctions for workforce members in violation of policies and procedures governing EPHI access or use
   - Termination of systems access
   - Session termination policies and procedures for inactive computer systems
   - Policies and procedures for emergency access to electronic information systems
   - Password management policies and procedures

- Secure workstation use (documentation of specific guidelines for each class of workstation (i.e., on site, laptop, and home system usage)
- Disposal of media and devices containing EPHI

b. Other Documents:
- Entity-wide Security Plan
- Risk Analysis (most recent)
- Risk Management Plan (addressing risks identified in the Risk Analysis)
- Security violation monitoring reports
- Vulnerability scanning plans
  o Results from most recent vulnerability scan
- Network penetration testing policy and procedure
  o Results from most recent network penetration test
- List of all user accounts with access to systems which store, transmit, or access EPHI (for active and terminated employees)
- Configuration standards to include patch management for systems which store, transmit, or access EPHI (including workstations)
- Encryption or equivalent measures implemented on systems that store, transmit, or access EPHI
- Organization chart to include staff members responsible for general HIPAA compliance to include the protection of EPHI
- Examples of training courses or communications delivered to staff members to ensure awareness and understanding of EPHI policies and procedures (security awareness training)
- Policies and procedures governing the use of virus protection software
- Data backup procedures
- Disaster recovery plan
- Disaster recovery test plans and results
- Analysis of information systems, applications, and data groups according to their criticality and sensitivity

- Inventory of all information systems to include network diagrams listing hardware and software used to store, transmit or maintain EPHI
- List of all Primary Domain Controllers (PDC) and servers
- Inventory log recording the owner and movement media and devices that contain EPHI

Evolution of State Health Information Exchange

Document released by The Agency for Healthcare Research and Quality (AHRQ), U.S. Department of Health and Human Services, and available at

[http://www.avalerehealth.net/research/docs/State_based_Health_Information_Exchange_Final_Report.pdf]

Dates of Note

2003: QHA established

2004: HIE Network launched

Overall Program Objective

Provide access to timely, reliable health information which will increase efficiencies, improve clinical outcomes, and lower costs.

Engaged Stakeholders

State Government

Physicians

Physician Associations

Hospitals

Business coalition

Health Plans

Employers

Consumers

Research Organizations

Vendors and Consultants

Target Population
Statewide

Technology/Infrastructure
CDR
EHR
eRx
Electronic Laboratory Reporting (eLab)
Unique Patient Identifier Number (UPIN)
Patient Portal
Employer Portal
Initial project—implement multiple applications in a small region

Funding
Initial member donations—$80,000 and in-kind support
Federal—$500,000
Subscription and data source fees
Data sales for research
Anticipated State and additional private sector funding

Timing
Implementation of EHR and CDR under way in select physician groups on Maui; roll out will continue in 2006 across physicians groups island wide and expand to neighboring islands in 2007 and beyond Unique Program and State.

Features
Heavy physician and business leader involvement
Large rural population with geographic disbursement
Health insurance mandate for all Hawaii employers
Consumer (patient portal) and employee wellness focus
AHRQ implementation grant recipient
Discounted single vendor solution

Overview

The Quality Healthcare Alliance (QHA), established in 2003, is a non-profit consortium of health care stakeholders and State and local government agencies in Hawaii whose vision is to transform health care to a patient-centered care model that will drive quality care. QHA recognizes the importance of providing information to the patient as a tool for managing health and understands that access to timely, relevant, reliable, and secure health information is the missing link in supporting patient centered care.

Timeline

2002—HBHC creates HIE model and writes businessplan

January 2003—HBHC joins with Hawaii Medical Association (HMA) and the Hawaii Independent Physicians Association (HIPA)

May 2003—HBHC, HMA, and HIPA hold Statewide conference crafting an agreement to build an HIE model measuring clinical outcomes; QHA established to implement

August 2003—QHA builds goals and clinical measures

September 2003—Measures adopted; QHA adds legislators, health plans, government agencies, labor unions, and regulators

2004—HIE network planning and collaboration development

2005–2006—Roll out to Maui

QHA's vision of a Statewide HIE network acts as a catalyst for transforming health care where quality and wellness, not illness, is the focus. The idea to create an HIE network actually dates back nine years, to a group of Hawaii physicians. At the time, these physicians were unable to garner support or a commitment from the necessary stakeholders, nor did they possess the business expertise to organize, build, or implement an HIE project. Years later, the business community came together with a shared vision for improving the health care system and a belief that costs could be effectively managed by focusing on quality. Toward this end, business leaders, technology experts, and physicians from the Hawaii Medical Association, the Hawaii Independent Physicians

Association, the Hawaii Business Health Council (HBHC)5, and the Medical Exchange of Hawaii formed QHA to transform health care in Hawaii through HIE. Notably, QHA recognized the importance of representing all market segments and spent its first year engaged in collaborative discussions across all major stakeholder groups, with an emphasis on including physicians. Since its inception, additional industry leaders, government agencies, and legislators have joined QHA. Its current Board includes a patient/consumer representative, and a Medicaid and a Medicare representative. As a result of its early outreach and collaborative efforts, QHA has engendered the support and trust of the business and health care communities. The HIE network and supporting infrastructure will be a CDR with interoperable EHRs accessible by the internet or a VPN that will capture and support exchange of clinical, administrative, and claims data. The systems will be flexible to allow interconnectivity and interoperation with stakeholders' legacy systems, as well as provide realtime access and reporting. The network will also support a patient portal and PHRs. Ultimately, QHA intends to target Hawaii residents Statewide although it currently separates its target population into three major segments: 1) employees and dependents of HBHC companies and labor union members covered by commercial health plans; 2) Medicaid population; and 3) Medicare eligible population.

SSL Handshake

The SSL protocol uses a combination of public-key and symmetric key encryption. The first step in any SSL session is the SSL handshake. The purpose of the handshake is to allow the server to authenticate itself to the client using public-key cryptographic techniques.

Server authentication requires the server to furnish a certificate whose contents are as shown below. It also needs the client (usually the browser) to have available details of the CA (Certifying authority) as indicated below.

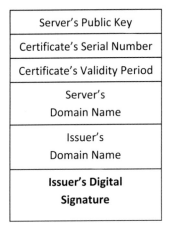
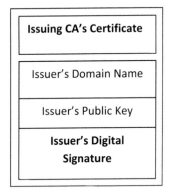

The Server authentication requires commences with the server providing o the client its certificate. The following steps are then performed.

a) The client verifies that the server certificate is within its validity period.

b) The client verifies that the CA who issued the server certificate is a trusted CA, i.e., the client has the certificate of the issuing CA.

c) The client verifies that the CA's public key validates the issuer's digital signature. To do this, it verifies that the public key from the CA's certificate (from its own list of trusted CAs) can validate the CA's digital signature in the server certificate that has been presented.

d) The client verifies that the domain name specified in the server's certificate matches the actual domain name of the server.

The server is authenticated if all the above steps execute successfully.

Subsequently, the client and the server undertake the exchange of symmetric key (called the session key) that is to be used for the subsequent encryption/decryption of two-way data communication during that session.

This happens as follows. Using all data generated in the handshake so far, the client (with the cooperation of the server, depending on the cipher being used) creates the premaster secret for the session, encrypts it with the server's public key (obtained from the server's certificate), and sends the encrypted premaster secret to the server. The server uses its private key to decrypt the premaster secret, then performs a series of steps (which the client also performs, starting from the same premaster secret) to generate the master secret. Both the client and the server use the master secret to generate the session keys, which are symmetric keys used to encrypt and decrypt information exchanged during the SSL session and to verify its integrity—that is, to detect any changes in the data between the time it was sent and the time it is received over the SSL connection.

Index